What
God Is
Honored
Here?

What God Is Honored Here?

Writings on Miscarriage and Infant Loss by and for Native Women and Women of Color

Shannon Gibney and Kao Kalia Yang Editors

UNIVERSITY OF MINNESOTA PRESS

MINNEAPOLIS

LONDON

Copyright 2019 by Shannon Gibney and Kao Kalia Yang

Individual essays and poems copyright 2019 by their respective authors

Published by the University of Minnesota Press
111 Third Avenue South, Suite 290
Minneapolis, MN 55401-2520
http://www.upress.umn.edu

A Cataloging-in-Publication record for this book is available from the Library of Congress.

ISBN 978-1-5179-0793-8 (pb)

Printed in Canada on acid-free paper

The University of Minnesota is an equal-opportunity educator and employer.

24 23 22 21 20 19   10 9 8 7 6 5 4 3 2 1

For the women in this anthology and women everywhere
who have experienced pregnancy loss, or whose babies have died.
For all we have lost, and all we love.

what have we come to now
what ground is this
what god is honored here

—*Lucille Clifton, "eyes"*
(quoting from The Gospel at Colonus)

Contents

Reclaiming Life

Shannon Gibney and Kao Kalia Yang

Miscarriage. Stillbirth. Neonatal loss. Fetal and infant death.

None of these words were new to us. We were writers. We were women. We were daughters. We were mothers, we were on our way to becoming mothers. And yet, our knowing the words could not prepare us for the experience of them. None of who we had been could have prepared us for who we would become in the wake of these words.

Grief is a lonely place we have all visited by ourselves, occasionally with others. Some of us have built homes to house our grief. Others shiver in the storms that break, unsure of where to hide, how to hide, whether they want to hide. Each of us, in our own ways and for many of us through our words, has encountered grief. All of us have awoken from despair only to find ourselves forsaken on its shores.

Six years after the loss of Baby Jules, a miscarriage at nineteen weeks, even in the years after when I, Kalia, had given birth to a living daughter and two living sons, I still feel the ghost of him swimming inside of me late at night and early in the morning when the world is quiet and dark. When the bigness of the sky enters through the window of our bedroom, when my husband is on his left side lost in his sleep, when behind the wall of our bed, I can make out the twists and turns of my sleeping children, my hands move high on my soft belly, so I can feel the force of life within me.

In the space of quiet possibility, Baby Jules moves inside of me, no longer as low as he had been. In fact, less than in my womb, he now swims close to my beating heart.

Four years after my first daughter, Sianneh, died inside me at forty-one and a half weeks, I, Shannon, feel her everywhere. She never made it into this particular world, but she made a home of me for nine long months, growing and becoming. Cradling her long, thin body in my arms after she was born, I had a new knowledge of how love can cleave you from the inside out, waiting, dreaming, hoping for a baby to take a breath who can never take a breath. Waiting for the truth to become something living.

There is no recovery from the loss of life's possibilities. We both tried, in our different ways, to make peace with what had transpired. I, Kalia, talked to my mother, who had been a warrior by my side through the work of bringing my quiet, transparent little boy into the world, a woman who had herself experienced seven miscarriages in her life. I, Shannon, spoke with my mother, who had been a neonatal nurse, caring for premature, sick, and dying babies for more than twenty-five years. Each of them, in their love for us, in the breadth and wisdom of their experiences, did what they could to try and piece together our broken hearts. We found solace and solidarity in our pain with our partners, our friends, and our communities. But it was the simple knowledge that we were not alone in the experience—we had never been and would never be—that taught us both that life would continue as if our babies had never lived if we didn't do something to commemorate their existence, all of their existences. Although we would never do the work of raising them, we had to raise ourselves, do the hard work of living in the absence of who they and we could have been together.

In the days, months, and years after, we both looked desperately for answers in medical studies, statistics, in literature, and in life for some response to our experiences beyond the immense loss. We were doing what we had been trained to do as writers: finding meaning in human experience.

We looked near and far, but there were no satisfying medical explanations in our cases. In America, miscarriage and stillbirths are classified into three broad categories: problems with the baby, such as birth defects and/or genetics; placenta or umbilical cord problems, an unsustainable exchange of oxygen and nutrients from a mother to her child and vice versa; or the health condition of the mother, things such as uncontrolled diabetes, high blood pressure, and/or obesity—all health factors that are linked to class and race in this country. Like most women who experience pregnancy loss, fetal death, and infant death, we received no explanations from the doctors for what had happened.

Like the medical explanations, the statistics were not helpful in explaining what happened to us. In fact, they troubled us further. According to the Centers for Disease Control (CDC), in the general population of the United States, 15 to 20 percent of pregnant women will experience a miscarriage in their lifetime, and stillbirths affect about 1 percent of all pregnancies. This means that each year about 600,000 women in America experience losses, and about 24,000 babies are stillborn. In 2015, the overall infant mortality rate was 5.9 percent for every 1,000 births. This is already a high rate for a rich, industrialized country such as the United States. But the numbers become even more disturbing when disaggregated by race. Again, according to the CDC, in 2015 infant mortality rates per 1,000 live births were 11.3 percent for black babies, 8.3 percent for American Indian babies, 5 percent for Latinx babies, 4.9 percent for white babies, and 4.2 percent for Asian American babies. In fact, according to the CDC, a risk factor for miscarriage and stillbirth is "being of the black race."

There is a growing body of research that confirms that the stress from racism that black mothers—and we can assume other women of color and indigenous women experiencing systemic oppression in this country—endure throughout their lifetimes makes it more difficult to carry their babies to full term. In a 2017 article for National Public Radio, "Stress from Racism May Be Causing African American Babies to Die More Often," Rhitu Chatterjee writes:

In 2004, [Richard] David [neonatologist at the University of Illinois, Chicago] and [James] Collins [Northwestern University Medical School] published a study in the *American Journal of Public Health* in which they reported the connection between a mother's experience of racism and preterm birth. They asked women about their housing, income, health habits and discrimination. "It turned out that as a predictor of very low birth weight outcome, these racial discrimination questions were more powerful than asking a woman whether or not she smoked cigarettes," David says. Other studies have shown the same results.

While the research is confirming what many of us women of color know about our bodies and our lives in a landscape where white supremacy's reach goes far and deep, it also points to the historical and ongoing medical research gender gap.

We know far less about women's health, including pregnancy, because women have been historically and persistently excluded from toxicology and biomedical research. Funding for studies focused on women's health issues in particular are few and far between. All of these issues are critical and must be tackled in earnest if we are to get to the bottom of disproportionate infant loss and miscarriage among women of color in this country, much less have any chance of changing it.

Furthermore, in a country that had 23,000 infant deaths in 2015, there is little to no public talk of these babies, their lives in the world or in utero, or the dreams of the families they carried with them. In many ways, for the mothers and families who lost these babies, the inability and lack of public space to talk about them are a second death. The silence makes us feel as if there is something fundamentally wrong with *wanting* and *needing* to remember our children, no matter how short their lives may have been. But if there is one lesson that has emerged from these tragedies, it is that our individual and collective healing is intimately bound up in the process of remembering them and us when we were with them, even if it means we must also remember and survive once again the moments when we lost them.

In that spirit, in the course of each of our journeys of loss, we looked to what we both love for answers: literature. Alas, all that we could find for grieving mothers was written by white women and often reflected only their experiences, and thus without thought or intention marked the disappearance of our own experiences as grieving mothers, as women of color. Where were the pregnancies like ours? Where were the babies like ours? Where were we in this world of longing?

After the loss of our pregnancies and babies, we both knew we wanted to write of our experiences individually, but we had a suspicion that we needed each other's strength to finish the work. Still, we couldn't get ourselves to the page because we were not yet ready, so we let the days turn into nights, the moon orbit around the earth, the earth orbit around the sun, and we watched our stories of motherhood change and each other grow in the changes. We both had more children. We both came to a place where we knew the children we had were the only ones we would give birth to. Our stories of our childbearing years were playing themselves out. Finally, five years after the loss of Baby Jules, and four years after the loss of Baby Sianneh, we were ready to be found, to find ourselves on the pages—with our fellow indigenous women and women of color.

As storytellers, we wanted to dive into and recuperate the narrative gap. We wanted the women and families who experienced fetal and infant death to be able to represent themselves and their particular truths. We wanted the babies who have been lost to become embodied and to discard their ghostly presence in the larger societal narrative. We, lovers of language, wanted to journey into the landscape of loss with other indigenous women and women of color and to return from it, with a token of what could and could not be delivered in the promise of motherhood, in the living and the dying that we go through as daughters, sisters, and mothers. This project is our claim on our lives as indigenous women and women of color who have experienced infant and fetal loss, in its many forms.

What we found through embarking on this project was each other: two women of color writers who had experienced gut-wrenching loss that was nowhere in the public discourse. Kalia, as a Hmong American writer and refugee, had written about the struggles of being Asian American in a white cultural context before but never in the context of herself as a mother. Likewise, being a mixed black transracial adoptee, Shannon had written about how blackness and gender intersect in her fiction and nonfiction, but somehow the role of mother and the experience of loss in this area hadn't made their way into her work. Both of us deeply respected each other's work and had a sense that we had the opportunity to create a much-needed space for expression, exploration, and connection between and among indigenous women and women of color who had lived through devastating loss. Once we fully committed to the project, we put out a call for submissions, and as we started sifting through the many incredible pieces we received, we began to realize that this work was healing *us,* and that we were healing each other.

The myriad women who courageously sent us their stories of unforeseen tragedy, of the often not-so-hidden racism and sexism of the medical establishment, of the small and sharp and sometimes even blunt words and actions of people after the fact that only made things worse, buoyed us and let us really feel the import and urgency of this work. Although their mode of expression was words, what they were really doing, what we were really doing, was expelling, processing, and addressing trauma. This was further reflected in the time revising that many of these women tirelessly put in to make their already resonant pieces stronger. "I'm sorry I'm behind schedule. This is harder to revisit than I thought," was a message we received often. "I just seem to sit in front of the computer and stare. I can't seem to get it out," was another. In response to an editorial note that we needed an author to slow down and linger in a scene longer, she said tearfully, "I just realized I wrote it like that because I didn't want to acknowledge how violent that experience was—the way the hospital staff treated me as a black woman. I didn't want to see that and feel that again." Throughout the course of a long winter, lit by the fires inside our wombs and our hearts, we journeyed together far and deep into ourselves, across generations of mothers and daughters, to deliver to each other our most honest, poignant, and precious experiences of miscarriage and infant loss.

For the two of us, holding and helping to shape these stories, creating a vessel to adequately carry them and share them with the world has been an honor and a privilege—one that we are so grateful for, as it has brought us much closer together both professionally and personally. There are not many stories of black and Asian American women coming together through loss in American popular culture, but we know through the process of putting this book together that our lives have been forever transformed by each other's. We experienced how indigenous women and women of color connecting through loss and storytelling can create lifelong friendships that anchor us and foster power and community among each other.

The title for this collection, *What God Is Honored Here?*, comes from Lucille Clifton's quotation of a lyric from *The Gospel at Colonus* in her poem "eyes," collected in her book *Quilting: Poems, 1987–1990*. Clifton, who herself experienced miscarriage and wrote of it beautifully in a piece called "the lost baby poem," which we share in the pages that follow, was no stranger to the faith and the fears of women and mothers. In the meeting of life and death, each of us, in our own separate worlds beneath our own separate skies, has asked the question, "What God is honored here?" When the doctor looks meaningfully at the lab technician and in the still cold of the air utters words that make no sense, still now, years later: "I'm sorry. The heart has stopped. Your baby is dead." When you ask yourself and those around you who are supposed to be medical experts what the best path, or any path, forward is, and there is no answer. Alone in your bedroom in the small hours of morning, the hollow in your belly growing with each inbreath, you may well ask the mute wall: "What God is honored here?" And what you may find, while reading through the stories contained here, is that paradoxically in your aloneness you were actually in community with women you couldn't see or hear but whose knowledge of loss lay as deep in their organs as their/your babies once did.

This anthology is a collection of voices from indigenous women and women of color who have experienced those words that so many of us were familiar with but only in the aftermath of what happened realized where their meanings live, words that now pause our hearts: miscarriage, stillbirth, neonatal loss, fetal and infant death. This is a collection with award-winning writers and poets as well as women who are first-time writers. These women are writing of matter that barely became babies, of babies that they carried for weeks and months, to term and past term, of complex medical procedures to remove "tissue," and of vaginal births. Some women's experiences are deeply intertwined with their cultural and spiritual backgrounds, while for others, these issues are immaterial. We raise our voices together, indigenous women and women of color from across the expanse of this country, across the generations of women, to speak to our experiences of miscarriage and infant loss not simply to fill a void but to build bridges of hope and healing from that void, to say to each other: we are *here*.

Here, where we are important and our children matter profoundly to us, in the space where they were and where they continue to be.

References

Chatterjee, Rhitu. "Stress from Racism May Be Causing African American Babies to Die More Often." NPR. https://www.npr.org/sectionshealth-shots/2017/12/20/570777510/how-racism-may-cause-black-mothers-to-suffer-the-death-of-their-infants. December 20, 2017. Accessed on April 1, 2018.

Danielsson, Krissi. "Making Sense of Miscarriage Statistics." VeryWell Family, March 21, 2018. https://www.verywellfamily.com/making-sense-of-miscarriage-statistics-2371721. Accessed on April 2, 2018.

"Infant Mortality." Centers for Disease Control. https://www.cdc.gov/repro
    ductivehealth/maternalinfanthealth/infantmortality.htm. Accessed on
    April 1, 2018.

"The Medical Research Gender Gap: How Excluding Women from Clinical Trials
    Is Hurting Our Health." *Guardian*. April 30, 2015. https://www.theguardian
    .com/lifeandstyle/2015/apr/30/fda-clinical-trials-gender-gap-epa-nih-institute
    -of-medicine-cardiovascular-disease. Accessed on April 1, 2018.

Quinn, Molly, and Victor Fujimoto. "Racial and Ethnic Disparities in Assisted
    Reproductive Technology Access and Outcomes." *Fertility and Sterility* 105,
    no. 5 (May 2016).

Statistics Brain. "Pregnancy Statistics." September 2016. https://www.statistic
    brain.com/pregnancy-statistics/. Accessed on April 2, 2018.

the lost baby poem

Lucille Clifton

the time i dropped your almost body down
down to meet the waters under the city
and run one with the sewage to the sea
what did i know about waters rushing back
what did i know about drowning
or being drowned
you would have been born into winter
in the year of the disconnected gas
and no car   we would have made the thin
walk over genesee hill into the canada wind
to watch you slip like ice into strangers' hands
you would have fallen naked as snow into winter
if you were here i could tell you these
and some other things
if i am ever less than a mountain
for your definite brothers and sisters
let the rivers pour over my head
let the sea take me for a spiller
of seas   let black men call me stranger
always   for your never named sake

Then and Then

Sidney Clifton

May 1989

I check in at the desk. Last name, first name: "Termination, first
trimester."
The facility is clean and small and prepared for protesters. In the waiting
room I shift into observation mode.
No heart, only data.
This is happening.
The girl and her boyfriend sitting across from me are maybe fourteen
years old. Her mother sits beside her, Not-Looking at the boy.
I'm alone. Strong. Brave. This is the right thing.
This is really happening.
My marriage is dead. We have two children. I do not need three.
I can do this. My mother did. Five times. My sister did. Three times.
This is really happening.

I'm wearing the gown (open in back), climb up on the table. The
machine to the left, doctor seated on a rolling stool by my feet.
Nurse near my right shoulder. She tries to be an angel. She is not.
All business, no heart; I need facts and data. "It's about two inches long

now, right?" I ask. Not-Angel chuckles. "Oh, it's a little bigger than that," she says. I swallow my shame instead of punching her. The doctor turns on the machine while numbing my cervix. My teeth and legs tremble.

"I'm cold," I say to Not-Angel. She replies, matter-of-fact, "It's not the cold, it's the tension. Everybody feels this way."

She needs to shut the fuck up.

No heart. Just data. No heart. Just data.

The machine turns on, sounding like a coffee grinder or a blender, something sharp that destroys things. Doctor asks, "Ready?" "Yep!"

I lie.

Doctor inserts the instrument and now everything is sound (no heart)

that gets louder (no heart)

and louder like a garbage disposal grinding too many scraps (no heart)

and (I'm sorry)

after (no heart) ten minutes (no heart)

finally finally finally (no heart)

it's all (no heart) over

(noooooooooheeeeeaaaarrttt)

It was the right thing.

It is the right thing.

I get dressed. Stand up straight, despite wearing a superduper absorbent maxi pad.

It was the right thing.

I pray my apology.

All heart.

Only heart.

I'm sorry, baby.

It's not your time.

Mommy loves you.

Please forgive me.

It's the right thing.
In my imaginings s/he understands.

March 2005

Knees up, legs open; OB-GYN doing a vaginal ultrasound. I peed on
a stick last week and got the faint double lines. The familiar "swish-
swish-swish-swish" when the techno-dildo finds the embryo (or is
it a fetus yet?) and I am more validated than joyous. Of course I'm
pregnant. And yes, I know I'm forty-five, but I come from a line of
Magic Mamas. I got this.
Six weeks earlier, we dropped off our daughter's crib at Goodwill. She
is in a big-girl bed now that she is three. I sighed, deep breath; equally
relieved, sentimental, and ready to get on with it. "I think I want another
one," he says, laughing. I jokingly grab him by the throat and pretend to
strangle him. We are laughing, but I don't know what this means.
My mind is a tornado and I can't grab onto any one feeling/thought/
image for any significant amount of time.
I would like our girl to have a sibling closer to her age but I am
just getting my body back. I love being pregnant: the process,
transformation, wonder, miracle. I hate leaving my baby to go back to
work. And I will have to go back to work . . . but wait, this could be a boy.
Our boy. His son.
I don't know what this means.

April

The script is different for pregnant women of Advanced Maternal
Age. We are the objects of concern, delight, and flat-out humor.
I'm not crazy, doctor. Just fertile. And I admit, basking in the "fuck you,
patriarchal pregnancy guidelines!" of it all.
Eat right, get exercise, rest when my body says so, and call the doctor if

I feel anything unusual. She says the usual stuff, except with a wry grin and a slightly shaking head.

What I think it means is that I am a badass, and we might have a son. My boy-obsession is a whirlwind and I already see him with his sister and his big big strong black brothers have to make sure he knows what it means to be a black man in America even with his white father make sure he values his blackness what do we decide about circumcision will this son make his father love me more is he a silently wished-for thing will his sister be a better big sister for a brother will he and his sister be friends after we are gone will he be brave be strong be beautiful be be be be?

May

We have just finished dinner and something is off. No nausea, no headache, but the vibrating like a tuning fork tapped firmly and held just so. The stillness is vibrating. The "I" of me is vibrating.

A trickle of fluid. I dash to the bathroom. Yellow fluid in my underwear. No. Nonononono rushing to my phone pretending to be calm.

"Something is wrong," I say in pretend while I wait for the doctor's answering service. I explain what has occurred in clinical, detached detail. My appointment is for the next morning. There is no pain, only vibrating and waiting.

Next morning at the doctor's office, another ultrasound. The just-turned-fetus (at ten weeks) is still. No heartbeat. I watch with clinical detachment as the doctor tries different angles but we both know and I say it first. "I don't hear anything." She concurs. Clinical Me crumbles. "Can you get my husband, please?" She brings him in and I am trying to be brave and trying to have Not Wanted This Baby So Much. I summon Clinical Me and am back at attention, next steps, how do we take care of this? We can wait for me to miscarry at home or get admitted to the hospital and have a D&C. I choose Option B.

The D&C the next day is comparatively easy. Go in, put on the paper
outfit, make jokes in the OR, go under, wake up.
Wait for results of the findings.
I need findings found.
I need to know what this means.

June

Finally an answer. Trisomy 13. "Incompatible with life."
But was it my son or daughter who was incompatible with life?
Until I know, I will not know what this means. Daughter means "not
another," "not this one," "you have already been blessed." Son means
"no boys for him" means "you have not earned him," means "you had
your chance and blew it."
My heart is a madwoman screaming. I don't know what this means.

Finally (eleven years later)

My OB-GYN retires. My entire Obstetric history is sent to me on a CD.
I scour every single page until finally, answers: Trisomy 13, XX. It was
a daughter we lost.
And then gained. One year later—2006—I birthed a healthy daughter.
She is strong. Beautiful. Smart. Brave. Brilliant.
We have been blessed.
I know what that means.

Lessons from Dying

Sarah Agaton Howes

I should have known that babies died, but in 2005, I did not.

I didn't know how to watch for the page turns. I remember the nurse's face when she looked at my ultrasound. I didn't know I could watch and analyze her face and see my daughter's death written all over her eyes. I didn't know that going straight to the hospital meant things were wrong and the sprinting nurse meant things were over.

I was five days past my due date with my first child. I didn't understand when the nurse said, "There is no heartbeat." I told the nurse to revive the baby.

It's not like I had lived a blessed life, but I hadn't known tragedy this way. My parents loved me, but I watched abuse and addiction around me my whole life. I thought I would be the lucky one. I didn't know yet that there are no lucky ones.

I didn't know that you had to go through labor to deliver your dead child. Our beautiful daughter Mahali Josephine was born August 31, 2005. She had long wavy hair and was "perfect in every way," according to the nurse, "except she's dead."

I carried her out of the hospital. The nurses thought we were delusional. But one thing about Anishinaabeg is we follow our own sets of rules. I knew there would be no explanations, no autopsies, no funeral homes. So I wrapped her up, they wheeled me out like the "real moms," and we drove her home.

Did you know you could keep your tiny baby this way? I stared at her for twenty-four hours to be sure there had not been a mistake. That she wouldn't suddenly gasp for breath. That this all wasn't some cruel hoax. Nothing. There was nothing left. I had no ceremony for this. I made things up. I gave her tiny moccasins and tiny special pajamas. Her grandpa made her a tiny box. We made up prayers and rituals and poured dirt over her tiny box. And then after a person buries their tiny baby in tiny moccasins in a tiny box, they are supposed to walk away from her.

I came home to a house full of baby clothes. Tiny diapers, tiny blankets, and bags of baby gifts lined the house.

After that, every movement felt slow and labored. And then I realized that I had also died. I couldn't breathe.

Losing your child is losing yourself. She died, I died. I didn't, I couldn't protect her. My body, what became known as the Death Trap had killed her. Or maybe the air had. The water? God? Who, who had killed my daughter?

A short list of what died that day: my daughter, me, my dreams, her future, all my gods, my laughter, the cabbage I covered my engorged breasts with, and this part of my stomach where I keep her sadness.

After 2005 I knew dead children were a thing. They became the only thing.

I built shrines and forts to her and all the other babies. Planted trees and burned things. I walked and cried to stones. All my dead gods continued their silence.

I had no songs, I knew no songs, I had no ceremonies, no gods. But there was a moment. I stood by a river, and I cried at the rocks. This sounds mystical, but in fact it was full of mosquitoes and mud and not romantic at all. But I got a song. It was really more of a call for help. It was me calling from the grave. Asking the mystery of this universe to help me. Please, please, please, please, please, please.

Everyone told us to wait to have another baby. But I became maniacal in my desire for another baby, any baby. Those crazed women who kidnap children began to make perfect sense to me. I told my husband to "give me another baby." I didn't care about anything else. Before I was even sure my body was healed, I decided to force my body into pregnancy again. My tiny baby number two didn't make it past month two. The Death Trap strikes again, I told them. My dead gods cursed me. Fuck the greeting card condolences and the meant to be bullshit, and all the optimism. All I had was death. And my song.

There was nothing for me but washing my hair. Washing the dishes. Dirty clean dirty clean. I stopped answering the phone.

Grief and total desperation joined me to so many women. My grand-mothers are the survivors of boarding schools, rapes, abuse, child abduction, and so much sadness. They surround me with their stories, their hands, their laughter, their bitterness, and their sheer determination to not die. I came from this legacy of sadness. But I also came from their legacy of survival. I came from their hardship. Without my knowing, I had prepared for this. I built them altars to add to the dead children altars.

I hated when people called me strong.

Against all sage advice, within the year, I was pregnant again.

I waited for this baby to die. Every day I waited for it. I fed the baby or-ange juice to make it move, went into rounds of endless ultrasounds, and somehow he survived. The Death Trap had produced a breathing, crying child who looked at me, and he saved me. My tiny Giniiwens flew over the world, saw my sadness, and came to bring me life. I decided to be a soldier to stand between death and my boy.

I wish I had been able to be better. But instead I just decided not to sleep. I watched him to make sure his chest rose and fell for eighteen months. I held him while he was asleep and awake. I kept our breathing in sync in this magical thinking way of making him stay with me. An owl, the messenger of death, perched itself out our communal bedroom. Every night I screamed at that goddamn owl. I told my husband to get rid of it or I was going to start shooting at it. But now, I wonder if that owl wasn't telling me that I was no longer dead either.

I never let this child out of my sight. Once on a plane the flight attendant offered to watch him so I could use the bathroom, and I said, "I don't know you!" She leaned in and said, "Ma'am, we're on a plane, where will I go?" But she didn't know that I was a soldier, and I dreamed magical thoughts, and I was terrified every day that my child was going to die.

But remember I had that song?

Repeatedly people in my community suggested I try ceremony, but my gods were dead, and I knew no ceremonies for this. I grew up a Christian-school, assimilated Indian girl and had become a dead assimilated one. But there was this little boy and his eyes. I wanted to be healthy for him, physically, spiritually, all the healthies. For him, I just went. I took a list of what I needed and went to ceremony. Alone.

There was not a magical moment where the lights shone down on me from the clouds. There was no mysticism. Through this searching, this desperate clawing at the grave to be alive enough to raise my boy, to meet his eyes, I found ceremony. My gods were dead but so were my ancestors, and so maybe I pray to them. Through this clawing I found so many beautiful people, and their love found me. Through this digging I found running and a community of women to surround me in running toward my life. Somehow through digging myself out of the grave, I realized it wasn't only me digging. This world offered life as much as death. Out of my deep sadness a hole had been dug out so deep I experienced joy in a way only the grieved can.

Every day when I see my children, I am again amazed that they are breathing and have survived another day. Trauma changed me forever. But now my heart so gouged, my heart so billowed, my heart so open can explode with love. My heart has depth I am certain grief gifted me.

It turned out there was a whole universe waiting for me. A world of ceremony, art, laughter, prayer, songs, and my ancestors. I died to get here.

April Is the Cruelest Month

Michelle Borok

It was in spring, six years ago, that I fell madly and deeply in love with Mongolia. When the landscape was brown, the winds were cold, and the steppes were littered with the bleached bones of livestock that couldn't survive the winter. I felt the first stirrings of a life I could live here.

In Mongolia, in a small northern city called Darkhan, I began to build a life unlike any I could have imagined in Los Angeles. It came with a long-distance love story, cultural clumsiness, a daunting language gap, and a new, expansive family. This life became transformative with the birth of my daughter, Terra, and becoming a wife to Aagii. Eight months after her birth in December, in August 2013, I learned I was due for another—a son this time. Terra and I were both born in the Year of the Dragon. Our son would be born in the Horse Year, like his father.

I kept the second pregnancy under wraps, particularly from friends and acquaintances overseas. I spared people social media updates about cankles, heartburn, and baby bump photos. In part, it seemed so repetitive. So little time had passed since my first pregnancy, things felt more normal than noteworthy.

The early part of the pregnancy progressed without much fanfare. We knew what to expect and did all the things we were supposed to do, but with less stress and constant concern. I took my vitamins, cut some vices, and went to far fewer doctor's appointments just to be measured, have my blood pressure checked, and be told that everything was fine.

We used the public health care system—it had helped us deliver one healthy child before at a cost of just a couple hundred dollars. There is very little diagnostic testing done in Mongolia during pregnancy compared to in the United States. There are blood and urine tests along the way, an excessive number of ultrasounds, and a mandatory chest X-ray. The X-ray is taken in a gigantic, Soviet-era, sci-fi chamber of doom. You walk your body, one that feels fragile for all the preciousness of your cargo, into a giant lead box that screams radioactivity. A few loud clangs, some lights, and a technician eventually lets you out again. Aside from the ominous X-ray machine, for the most part, these screenings were fairly passive. My OB-GYN mostly looked for big red flags, not troubling points of light in the distance. We confidently started planning for life as a family of four with two under two.

There were no concerns until January. One night, I was struck with a sharp, relentless lower abdominal pain. It was unbearable, and my first concern was the baby. A late-night call to the doctor who delivered Terra had her at our apartment within ten minutes. An ambulance (a Russian jeep with a first-aid kit inside) arrived soon after, and the driver helped my husband and his cousin carry me down five flights of stairs to crawl into the backseat of our own car.

In the emergency room, the initial diagnosis was appendicitis, and the plan was immediate surgery for removal. After an ultrasound to make sure that the baby wasn't in any distress, my doctor came into the operating room to oversee the procedure. Once I was opened up, it was determined that the pain was the result of an ovarian cyst and not a ruptured appendix, so I was told the cyst would be removed instead. As the hole in my side was being stitched closed again, a nurse showed me a crimson and black mass the size of a small orange, before it was unceremoniously dropped into the biological waste bin.

I recovered from the surgery in the women's and maternity ward of the hospital, so that my doctor could monitor the health of the baby. I healed well and was back home within a week.

My belly kept growing. Into the eighth month, just weeks before the anticipated April eighteenth due date, it was time for another visit to the OB-GYN at the general hospital. My husband and I were instructed to see the ultrasound specialist down the hall from the OB-GYN's office. We had never seen her before, we'd always had them done at the private clinic on the other side of town, but it seemed important to be done then and there.

The hallway stretched the whole length of the hospital wing, lined with exam rooms for doctors of all kinds. It was packed with people that day, people who didn't want to step aside to let you pass, lest they lose their place in line to see a specialist. Nervous about the OB-GYN's insistence on the ultrasound that day, I gripped Aagii's hand tightly as he cleared a path to the exam room at the opposite end of the hall.

The ultrasound technician was abrupt and curt, in true Mongolian public service fashion, and told us that we were wrong about the baby's due date. She insisted that the baby was due in May and not April, as it only measured at thirty-one weeks of growth and development. When we repeated the date of my last menstrual cycle, she said we were wrong and told us to go report back to our OB-GYN.

We left the office in shock. There was clearly something wrong, and it wasn't our due date. There was something wrong with the baby. Foiled by one of Darkhan's frequent power outages, we went to our regular ultrasound specialist the next day for a second opinion.

Our regular specialist helped us understand what we were faced with. The baby had only two vessels instead of three in his umbilical cord, a condition that often affects fetal growth and development. Our baby was measuring far behind the standard for thirty-seven weeks of development. Although my girth had expanded, he said, I had more amniotic fluid than baby, which was something to be concerned about. He also saw an irregularity in the baby's left hand, indicating radial dysplasia, more commonly known as club hand. He suggested we see a doctor soon for more information. We made immediate plans to get consultation from doctors at Ulaanbaatar's First Maternity Hospital, the largest care facility in the country.

Our friend Bilegee came with me and Aagii to Ulaanbaatar to help translate at the hospital. Bilegee was an English teacher in Darkhan who befriended me when I first arrived in 2012. Her English was strong enough to help me navigate my new environment beyond what I could manage on my own with a Mongolian-English dictionary and Aagii's very limited English. However, she lacked the skills of a truly effective translator, editing at her own discretion. In addition, our friendship was superficial, usually involving reimbursement for services rendered.

We first went to the pediatric ward, since Bilegee said she had a friend there who was a doctor that would help us navigate the system. Half of Mongolia's entire population lives in Ulaanbaatar, and it's where most of the state's essential services are located. The First Maternity Hospital operates far beyond its capacity and is consistently understaffed and overworked. During the height of cold and flu season, the hallways of the hospital are lined with bedding parents have brought from home to share with their children for inpatient care.

After pushing our way through the crowded halls of the pediatric ward, we found ourselves in a section of the hospital for seriously ill children. We were told to wait on a bench in a hallway while Bilegee tried to contact her friend. For a half an hour we sat waiting. In front of us was a parade of children who were living with birth defects, tumors, and crippling disease. Aagii and I sat in silence, holding hands. We'd give each other a squeeze as the children passed by, sometimes joining us to sit on the bench. Every beautifully flawed child that walked past us felt like a preview. It was the first of the most tangibly difficult moments in our pregnancy, and it was ominous.

It was a difficult and long couple of days in UB. We met with a doctor who spoke English and seemed to have a good grasp of what needed to be done to get us answers. The doctor consulted with the hospital's top ultrasound specialist, and the senior doctors were presented with my case in their staff meeting, to arrive at a course of action. It was confirmed that the baby had club hand in at least one arm and that his growth was significantly delayed. They suggested that we postpone delivery only by one week, to give him extra time to grow safely.

An extensive echocardiogram was conducted, with several pediatric specialists looking on, and we were told that his heart was small, but it was functioning normally. With two weeks still left to go before his new due date of April 23, the doctors said that it would be fine for me to return to Darkhan with a plan to return to UB for a scheduled C-section. The neonatal care, which would likely be required, would be more extensive at the First Maternity Hospital. It would be challenging and expensive to give birth far from home, but we thought first of what our newborn son would need.

The following week we focused on getting the house ready for the baby. I sorted out his clothes, new ones from his grandparents and hand-me-downs from friends, and made space for him in Terra's room. I started researching noninvasive therapies for treating club hand and tried really, really hard not to get focused on the other complications that were often present for babies with the same diagnosis. We kept a bag of his things packed for the trip to UB and tried to relax and enjoy the downtime we had before life was going to change forever.

The next Monday, we went back to our regular ultrasound specialist to check on the baby and see if there had been any growth since he'd last been looked at. The doctor was concerned. The baby hadn't grown, and he seemed lethargic. He was a much more mellow baby than Terra was during my pregnancy, and while I knew he was much smaller than she had been in her final weeks in the womb, I chalked up the slowdown in movement to the normal slowdown of when their arrival is coming. In addition to the lack of growth and decreased activity, the doctor said that I had less amniotic fluid than the last time he had seen me. He felt that all of these things were problematic. We contacted all of the doctors we had consulted along the way, in UB and in Darkhan, but no one seemed especially alarmed. We carried on, concerned, but without many options. In the next couple of days, I spent quieter moments by myself thinking about how I would cope with losing the baby at this stage. As soon as those thoughts would come together, I'd scold myself for thinking negatively and force myself to try to remember the sound of his heart beating.

On Thursday we went in for another ultrasound. His heartbeat was gone.

My amniotic fluid was nearly gone, and the baby was dead. The technician asked when I had last felt movement, but I had felt something the night before. I was still feeling movement at that point, but it wasn't him, and I couldn't remember the last time I had felt something that couldn't be confused with mild contractions of my uterus. I don't remember much about that day, besides crying in the hallway of the hospital and walking from one end of it to the other to talk to the OB-GYN about what we had just learned. I remember Aagii's tears and then his resolve. He instantly became completely focused on my health, while I was crippled by the news.

After consulting with every doctor we had spoken to during the pregnancy, we were advised to go to the hospital the next day to deliver the baby. I repacked my bags for the hospital, with only a swaddle cloth for the baby. I went to sleep cradling my dead belly, which seemed heavier than ever.

The brief research I had done online suggested that a vaginal birth was the healthiest way for a mother to deliver a stillborn child, but I had had a C-section with Terra, and I was under the impression that I would have to have a second C-section. But we felt helpless and trusted in the doctors to know which course of action was the best to take.

On Friday morning we drove to the hospital. Bilegee joined us to help translate. We met with the head doctor at the maternity hospital, who had quickly consulted with the other doctors. She said that I would be checked in that morning and that on Monday, the doctors would decide whether I should give birth vaginally or have a C-section. That meant I would spend three days in the hospital, isolated from Aagii, Terra, and my family, lying on a bed in an active maternity ward with a dead baby inside of me. I insisted on knowing why that would be necessary. The doctor said that they would use those three days to monitor me and give me antibiotics. I insisted that if nothing was going to be done for three days, I be allowed to spend that time at home with my family. The doctor said that was fine, but that if I had any problems or bleeding, to come to the hospital right away.

I had no problems or bleeding, just the odd contraction now and then, my body trying to move on. I spent the next three days with the people I loved, trying to prepare myself emotionally for what I was about to go through. I also tried to learn what I could about what the experience would be like, or at least what it was like in American hospitals. Good friends rallied for me and offered tremendous amounts of love and support while I was still operating in a fog of despair and disbelief. I spent three days trying to ignore my reflection in the mirror, the continued contractions, and the kind but careless touches of my belly by concerned family members. I still felt "pregnant" while the baby was still inside me, but I understood that I was giving birth to the death of a dream.

On Monday we returned to the hospital. I was prepared to set limits about what would happen and to push for things I wanted to make the experience less awful. Monday ended up being a repeat of Friday. The doctor said that they would give me labor induction medication, but that it would take up to seventy-two hours for delivery. That gave me three more days with my dead son inside of me, which I was unhappy about. I asked again why surgery wasn't an option, and they insisted that vaginal birth was still the safest route for me. I made it crystal clear that I was un-happy about the length of time they were proposing, and that so few options were being presented, but there was nothing I could do. Over the weekend, Aagii and I had talked about going to UB for the delivery, but I was anxious about the idea of being far from our support network and then having to do the three-hour drive home with our dead son in the back seat of the car. We stuck with delivery in Darkhan, despite our apprehensions.

The first day in the hospital, I was angry and depressed and would cry periodically. I cried when I heard the baby in the next room crying and was reminded that I'd never hear my baby boy cry. When we had found out the baby wasn't well, I had felt guilty for feeling healthy and normal during the pregnancy. I lay in my hospital bed believing that the suffering I was finally experiencing was my punishment for being oblivious to the suffering of my son. I deserved what was happening for letting my son's life slip away without a fight, without even knowing he was lost to us.

The night nurse came around at midnight to check on all the patients and distribute medication. She checked my blood pressure and then pulled out an aluminum cone to listen for my baby's heartbeat. I lifted my nightgown to let her look, thinking surely she must be listening for some-thing else and knew there wasn't a heartbeat to be listened to. She looked perplexed after her search, and then moved on to check on my roommate. After she was finished with the mother with the living child, she told me to follow her into the room across the hall. She wanted to use the fetal heartbeat monitor. As she was turning it on and waiting for it to boot up, I finally broke down and told her, in my broken Mongolian and tears, that there was no heartbeat for her to listen to. I left the room with heaving sobs and curled up into a ball on my bed.

The next day, I started receiving induction medication. The contrac-tions increased in frequency but not in severity, and dilation proceeded very, very slowly, by fractions of a centimeter. In the afternoon, Aagii brought Terra to the hospital for a visit. I sneaked out of my room to go outside to see them. I was reminded of why I needed to stay strong; I had a living child who needed me. About an hour after their visit, the contractions began in earnest. They grew from tingling discomfort to increasingly unbearable, gut-wrenching pain. I was completely unprepared for what the physical experience of labor would be like. The worst moment came when I felt the churning and locking into place of what felt like solid bone across my lower abdomen. I knew that the baby had been shifted into a horizontal position and that it would take another serious contraction to change that. I decided then and there that I would need pain intervention to survive another contraction of that magnitude.

Bilegee came to the hospital (after hanging up on two of my frantic calls) and spoke with the doctors. She told me that they said I couldn't have pain medication. She emphasized that all women who give birth experience this pain and that I needed to be patient and calm. She added that she had given birth to two babies, and she knew it was painful, but that I had to suffer through it. I asked her if she'd ever given birth to a dead baby, which quickly ended that conversation. I kept insisting on pain medication, reminding everyone that my dead baby wasn't going to be put at risk if I were to take it.

Bilegee told me that the doctors had asked that I "stop howling," at which point my "howling" turned into heaving sobs as I curled up into the smallest ball I possibly could, bleeding into an adult diaper that wouldn't stay on and pounding my head and fists against the wall. While motherhood is celebrated in Mongolia, it turns out that women are expected to go through labor in silent stoicism. Vocal expressions of their pain are reprimanded. In the older, Soviet-era public hospitals, women in the final stages of labor are strapped into chairs with wrist restraints.

Eventually, the doctors agreed to let me have an epidural with a catheter. The anesthesiologist tried to administer it as I sat backwards on a wooden chair from the nurses' station. I tried to stay as still as possible while the contractions continued. He jammed needles into my lower back three times, and on the fourth attempt, my right leg violently spasmed and a painful, burning sensation ran from my toes to my hips. He tried again, with the same painful result, this time with the pain spreading farther across my hip to my left leg. At this point, now terrified that I was going to be left with debilitating nerve damage or paralysis, I yelled for the procedure to stop.

Nothing more happened that night. The pain of my contractions continued, but I tolerated it. I vomited a few times and used a bedpan because it was too painful to walk down to the end of the hall to use the single toilet shared by all the patients on the second floor. My dilation was checked and still far from progressing. Bilegee ended up spending the night in the now-vacated bed in my room. No more induction medication was given.

In the morning, the doctors gathered after an exam that showed little progress in dilation. Bilegee roughly translated what they had concluded. They said that if I were a Mongolian woman, they would have made me wait four weeks for my body to expel the baby on its own, but because I was a foreigner, they had been willing to try induction. They said that the induction was unsuccessful, and it was dangerous to try to deliver vaginally because my previous C-section scar might rupture. It was time to consider a second C-section to deliver the baby.

In my exhaustion, pain, and frustration, I found room for anger again. The doctors knew all along that I had had a previous C-section. Why had I been put through the process of "labor" if that process was risky from the beginning? There was no possible way for the baby to be safely delivered vaginally, as he was in a transverse position. I understood that a C-section carried risks as well. But there was no new danger. The baby had been dead for at least a week, and there were problems that could arise during surgery. Bilegee spoke with the doctors about those complications but wasn't translating anything for me. I caught bits and pieces on my own, mostly about bleeding out. I asked if they had blood for a transfusion if it was needed. Bilegee asked and was told they had "some."

Again, I was powerless. There were no other options but C-section, so I pushed the conversation forward. Schedule the surgery, and end this.

Aagii spoke with the doctors after the conversation they had with Bilegee. He and cousin Jagaa came to my room. Jagaa and Aagii had tears in their eyes, and the color was gone from Aagii's face. He had heard the information about the risks and was terrified. Their tears brought out my own. I asked Bilegee to tell me what the doctors had told them. She said, "There are so many risks, I can't tell you." Outside, in the parking lot, more family had gathered. They stood beneath my hospital room window with Terra. They prayed for me. Earlier that morning, the family monk had been called to our house for prayers and blessings with my family. They called out their love and concern for me and through their own tears, told me to be brave. I was moved beyond words. The anger left and was replaced by a resolute sadness that I was giving over my life, Terra's and Aagii's future, and facing the end of our lives with our son. I had no fight left in me but to stay whole for Terra.

I climbed the stairs to the third floor, where the surgery would take place, tears still flowing. I wasn't told to stop crying by the doctors anymore, just guided through getting undressed and into a hospital gown. A numbness kept growing inside me, and I composed a mantra to get me through the surgery: Get him out. Stay alive. Make sure Terra has a mom.

The baby was delivered sometime between 11:30 and 12:15, but I had no idea exactly when, since the doctors and nurses hardly spoke through the procedure. Extra cloth had been held up in front of me to keep me from seeing what was happening, and of course, there was the silence of a dead baby leaving the womb instead of the sharp cries of a living one.

As I watched the clock on the monitor beside me, I waited for the tugging I remembered when I was sewn back together after Terra's birth. Instead there was suctioning and discussion between the surgeons. Bilegee was waiting out in the hallway, and I yelled out for her to come in and tell me what was happening. The doctors said that my uterus had taken a beating and needed to come out, along with my cervix. They said they could sew me up and that I could get the hysterectomy later, or they could do it right then. With no particular desire to have a scalpel anywhere near me again in the future, I stared up at the ceiling—not fully processing what this new development meant—and said, "Fine."

Early on in the pregnancy, I had told Aagii that this was going to be our last baby. I didn't feel like being pregnant again, and two kids seemed like plenty for us, even if we were short on having the five we were instructed to have on our wedding day. One of each, a boy and a girl. We felt blessed. Terra was our little dragon (like Mom), and her brother was going to be our little horse (like Dad). It was as perfect a scenario as we could hope for. Even when we found out the baby wouldn't be perfectly healthy, we worried and were scared of what that would mean for us, but we wanted him here. The news of his health challenges had us even more resolute about not having another, and when he died, the thought of going through an entire pregnancy and losing a child a second time absolutely killed me. Now the choice was being taken away from me. Whether we wanted one or not, we would never have another child together again. I cried for yet another loss as the anesthesiologist prepared a general anesthesia, and I woke up six hours later in my recovery room.

When I came to, I found Aagii sitting on the bed across from mine. I had been dressed while I was out, and my legs were working again. I was given some morphine to ward off the pain, and my head felt fluffy, floaty, and out of focus. I had a catheter in me and a drainage tube coming out of my incision. It felt unreal to be lying there with the baby truly gone. I told Aagii that I still needed to see the baby. Bilegee had taken two cell phone photos of him before they cleaned him up. I could clearly see his arms. The club hand was evident in both of his hands, and his head was badly misshapen, most likely from the pressure of labor in an unforgiving womb, but I could see that he had a full head of black hair like Terra had when she was born. I wanted to know what color his eyes were, but they were closed in the photo. Aagii was worried about me seeing him but understood that it was something I needed to do. He spoke with the doctors, who said they would bring him the next day.

Aagii was able to stay with me in the room for two more days, as I was unable to get up and do things for myself. He was with me when they brought the baby in. The nurses had swaddled him in the blanket we brought. He was only there for a moment. He didn't look like a sleeping baby, he looked like a dead one, and I didn't ask them to linger, or try to hold him. It's not something I regret yet, but I may someday.

Later that day, the hospital conducted an autopsy. In addition to the club hand, the baby had a one-centimeter hole in his heart, and his kidneys were fused together. On top of his small size, he would have faced significant challenges if he had been born alive. Somehow, this news helped. Before we knew what he had been dealing with, I tried to comfort myself with the idea that he had died in a place of safety and security and that he was spared the trauma of birth and his first days spent in a plastic box with tubes inserted in him. It's still impossible to imagine that he didn't feel any pain or fear, and that continues to haunt me, but I can't undo what happened to him. I can't explain or understand why he, of all the babies brought into the world, was chosen to experience this. While I understand that guilt is a useless emotion and there's nothing that I did (or didn't) do to bring his problems on, it's still the first place my mind goes. As I lay in that room with Aagii, I continually apologized to him for losing our son. He made me stop. He was trying to move beyond our guilt and was looking to the responsibility held by the doctors we consulted with throughout the pregnancy, and the doctors who handled the delivery.

Our son is buried now, and the process of moving forward—slowly, cautiously, and continually looking over our shoulders—has begun. I'll have more to share about that someday, but this is the story of how our son came into this world and quietly left it. The story of how he is absent from our lives is ongoing. For the sake of his soul, we have to let go, but we're struggling. We stay focused on our daughter now. We feel incredibly lucky to have her, in light of what we lost and how we lost it.

A few days after our son's funeral, we heard about another couple who had lost their child at the same hospital. The baby was large, four kilograms, and the mother was having a difficult labor. The doctors—the same ones who attended to me—held off on giving her an emergency C-section, and the baby suffocated and died. The parents were devastated. They had a healthy baby who died because of the ambivalence of the maternity hospital doctors. It was a crushing story to hear. Again, it made us grateful for Terra, but our hearts broke all over again at the news. The anger rose again as well. There's no conceivable reason why women should continue losing their children this way, or be put through the nightmare of saying good-bye in the way I did.

My story isn't one about giving birth to a "sleeping" angel who will be present in our lives like a welcome ghost. He's not ever going to be forgotten, but we want him to be able to move on peacefully. In Mongolian Buddhist tradition, which embraces an afterlife that promises rebirth, I hope that the life my son had was as short as it was to give him a quick and painless passage into a better, healthier, and happier life.

Not Everything Is a Patch of Wildflowers

Maria Elena Mahler

Hallelujah, I screamed to my insides. Everything was going according to plan. But for some reason, after the intern rolled the gel over my tummy a few times, he left the room. He returned much later with another expert, who pushed the gel even harder. Without a word, they wheeled me into one of the private emergency rooms and left me there. My husband, Jacques, asked me for permission to go outside. I was sure he had to smoke. I waited and suspected that something must not have been right, since the gynecologist in charge didn't come and give me the results of the ultrasound. I was getting more attention than I really wanted. Nurses came in and out. One placed an IV in my arm per the instruction of Dr. Schott.

Dr. Schott eventually showed up with a sweet smile under his moustache, reminding me of an uncle doctor I had in Chile—the one who took my appendix. I liked him immediately, although his news was not so good.

"The ultrasound shows that you have an ectopic pregnancy, and from that place on the tube the embryo cannot develop and go full term. It's dangerous. It can create all kinds of complications and health risks to you, my dear."

He must have been speaking in another language. I could barely make out that my plans had to change. After only the gods know how long, his eyes stayed glued to mine, and all I could see was my uncle doctor in Chile. I nodded at his green lagoon eyes until he repeated:

"Do you understand?"

"Yes. I think so. What are my options?"

Jacques stood next to my bed and held my fingers tightly in absolute silence.

"You have two options," the doctor said with a sweet and knowing tone. "The first one is we perform a D&C, and for that we need to schedule you for surgery tomorrow. You can start bleeding any minute. Or the second option is we give you an injection that will terminate the pregnancy, and you will be good to go."

Still in disbelief I asked, "And what is in the shot? How do you know it's working?"

"You think we can leave next month to Mexico?" Jacques whispered in my right ear.

Like in a spell, I was tangled and slowly drowning in the doctor's familiar eyes.

"If you were in my shoes and had to choose between those two options, which one would you choose?"

Dr. Schott took another step closer to my bed. Taking the palm of my hand between his cupped hands, he said: "If you were my daughter, I would suggest you get the injection. First, it is quick and practically painless. Surgery, on the other hand, has a fifty-fifty chance of things going wrong."

"What's in the injection?" My guts cramped with anticipation.

"It's called interferon. It stimulates the immune system to go after the embryo and then dissolves it. You will resume bleeding like a normal period, and it will be over."

"And after the shot, I won't see you again? I'm all done?" I asked with a smirk on my face, trying to put all this inside a black box called nightmare, and hoping that all of a sudden I was going to wake up and be on the road to Puerto Ilusión, crossing with the geese over borders into Mexico and to the bed-and-breakfast we owned.

"I'll see you in four weeks after the injection. You can take a couple of days to think and talk with your husband, but no more than two. Before your next bleeding, in three to four weeks, we will do another ultrasound to make sure that everything is all right, and you guys can be on your way to Mexico." He said the last words looking at Jacques.

Jacques nodded and smiled under his moustache, not really knowing what to say. From his point of view, the quicker we got done with this the better.

The decision was clear. Option two was the fastest and sounded the easiest, not to mention the less traumatic to the body. It was definitely better than being put out and having some doctor scrape my uterus walls and sticking who knows what into my ovarian tube. The decision was as clear as the IV that kept dripping into my veins.

I told Jacques I wanted the injection.

"Now?"

"Yes. That way we can leave for Mexico in a month.

Fifteen minutes later, a nurse came in with a large syringe with interferon, and quickly it ran through my veins.

"Out of sight, out of mind" was another saying I learned from my years with Jacques. This time it applied perfectly. We pretended nothing had happened, and we went back home to make our normal preparations for our trip back to the sunshine.

Our two-year-old was standing with both hands on the window. From the car I gave him a big forced smile. And after a game of hide-and-seek, I avoided any playtime or talks about having a baby sister or brother.

A few days before our departure to Mexico, I had my final appointment with the doctor. Before seeing Dr. Schott, I was again lying on the table with the ultrasound specialist rubbing that fishy gel on my tummy, and like déjà vu he left the room again—abandoning me. My mind wanted to go to the worst places. A second ultrasound technician came in a few minutes later, and again he pushed the gel around and deeper into my belly in order to confirm the report. He sealed the envelope and told me to follow him to see Dr. Schott.

When I entered the doctor's office, he was just opening the results.

"Sit, please." He pointed to a row of gray chairs. I sat against the wall on the same side as his desk. On the wall in front I could read all of his Canadian credentials. I trusted him and was consoled that in four more days I would be on my way to Mexico, and all of this would be left buried on the outskirts of Thunder Bay with his blessing today. *Adieu.*

While he read the report, he kept comparing it with the earlier ultrasound pictures.

"Oh my God!" He used one hand to cover his wide-open mouth. He then rubbed his hand over his balding head, trying to bring some circulation to his brain. "I can't believe it. I made a mistake," he said with his voice almost breaking. "The baby was healthy and implanted in the walls of your uterus all along. The first reading was not so clear. You were only a couple of weeks pregnant then. This new one shows it was okay. It's still there where it is supposed to be."

As I listened to his voice, huge tears spilled onto the carpet. I wasn't sure what the feeling was that came up so strong, melting me into an avalanche. I couldn't tell why I cried. Maybe it was his honesty that touched my heart like the *cantaora* does with her sincere voice in flamenco. Or were these tears of happiness since now I could go on with my pregnancy? I could come back to Ontario after the winter and have the baby in spring. Through the flood of tears, I finally uttered:

"What does this mean? Can I have my baby now? You just said so, right?"

"No. We need to end your pregnancy before it's too late."

"Too late for what? I don't understand."

My head began to look for the exit of my labyrinth, and his words started to sound slower, like they were coming from deep underwater.

"You cannot have this baby." He could barely say the words. "If you are lucky enough to make it to term, the child will most likely be born with some deformity. Interferon can cause all kinds of problems, serious birth defects, three legs or two heads. Do you understand?"

My tears only understood the desire to roll down to the deepest part of some well.

"Malformation is really common in these cases," he insisted. "Besides, it's dangerous for you too. You could abort the baby any day, and you might not realize it. The fetus could stay inside of you and putrefy, poisoning your blood. I can't believe I made a mistake. Now we have to do the D&C. I'm going to schedule it for you at six thirty tomorrow morning."

I stood up in the middle of my puddle on his office floor so I wouldn't drown in myself.

"It's okay, doctor. We all make mistakes. Really, it's okay." I reached toward him in an impulse to give him a hug but had to slowly take it back.

I drove home in a trance, not believing what had just happened. I couldn't find the words to communicate the news to Jacques. How could I explain to my little angel that I was going to kill her the next morning? I had already honored her death, and now I had to go through it again.

Jacques didn't say much other than, "Sorry this happened," while he gave me a hug. He left me alone most of the afternoon. At least he had the good sense to know I needed some space. He watched cartoons with Sebastian, ate pretzels, and left the crumbs on the couch.

Tomorrow, the guillotine will spill blood down my walls, was all I could think. Then my heart would remember the doctor's pain—and my heart would cramp when I thought about him.

"You know we can sue him?" Jacques said before he began snoring that night.

The thought of lawyers and going to war made me feel worse. Making someone pay for their unintentional mistake wasn't going to change what happened. What is the point of revenge? To get satisfaction by seeing someone in as much pain as me? Wasn't he already in hell, feeling responsible like a father toward his daughter?

That night all the questions spanned out and collapsed into one vivid dream. I heard the owl on the cedar tree and the sound of snoring, then slipped into another reality as clear as the one I was just in. I was in the presence of Dr. Schott. We didn't speak. We just stood in front of each other and experienced an immense feeling of connection for one another. There were no colors other than white around us and no sound. We didn't need our eyes to see each other. We deeply felt each other. It was a most inexplicable soul-to-soul recognition. I spent most of my dream night with Dr. Schott.

Dawn was not welcoming for the unborn and the nameless. The early rays were weak and filtered through the few leaves left on the poplars. *Soon everything will die.* The only way to get through the long drive to the hospital was to feel the pain—not mine but his. His pain, his mistake, his repentance, his admittance, his fault, and his face were all that got me to the hospital without stopping along the highway and starting to vomit.

My legs were tight and crossed as I lay on a rolling bed wearing a light-blue paper robe. My curls hid in remorse inside the blue cap. I stared at the ceiling made of cheap white foam and at the green fluorescent lights. I prayed in vain for the nurse not to shave me. When she was done preparing me, I was left alone in a hallway by some door with a sign that read *Only Authorized Personnel.*

My heart skipped when I heard the echo of heels growing louder through the solitary hallway. When I tilted my head to see who was coming, I saw his grand figure walking toward me.

"I know I'm not supposed to see you. But I needed to see you." His voice was quiet and quick, and his face, with a mask hanging around his neck, got closer to mine. "I needed to tell you that last night you were with me all night." He placed his hand on his heart, and I could see his eyes water behind his glasses.

"I know, I know," I barely uttered. "You were with me too."

Dr. Schott and I smiled, and no more words were needed.

With an empty womb and dried tears, I woke up to my son's kisses.

"Wakee, wakee," Sebastian said, trying to wake me like I woke him some mornings. His soft cheeks felt tender on my face, and his hair tickled my lazy eyes. I could barely open them. I was still in and out of the anesthesia. I could feel a deeper level of the duality of this world, this plane, other planes, and how their borders can shape-shift. One can easily get lost in the net of Neptune, unable to distinguish one water from the other, and forget where we are.

After a week, we were able to leave for Mexico. I hoped that in that reality of sunshine, music, and beach, I could relearn to smile.

Tilted Uterus

When Jesus Is Your Baby Daddy

Taiyon J. Coleman

> 'bacca money
> so we thought to do better by ourselves
> to begin our next row
> we would go and get him
> because he was medically degreed in baby bringing
> because he was young and white and handsome
> and because of that
> had been neighbor to more knowledge
> there in the city
> than us way back behind
> the country's proud and inferior lines
>
> — *"The Afterbirth, 1931,"*
> *Nikky Finney*

It was the summer of 2000, and my pregnancy was considered high-risk because my OB-GYN diagnosed me with uterine fibroids. I woke from a deep sleep feeling period-like cramps in my stomach and my mattress shaking. I slept that night with my head at the foot of my single bed, which both my well-mannered grandmother and superstitious grandma would not have liked. Grandma always said that you should never sleep with your feet closer to your bedroom door than your head. She said it was very rude to let the bottoms of your feet be the first thing that greeted Spirits if you were so lucky to be graced with a visit from the dead during the night. Sleeping with my head at the foot of my bed was the only position where my pregnant body could feel the muggy August Iowa air being pulled into the hot and humid basement apartment by my cheap Walmart window fan.

At almost twenty weeks pregnant, the smell of everything made me disgustingly sick. It seemed that I could smell and taste someone eating a banana from a mile away. My boyfriend with Jesus's name, Emmanuel, was working a night shift at Krispy Kreme and wouldn't be home until well after midnight. When Emmanuel came home from work, I regularly made him take off his uniform and shower before he was allowed to enter our bedroom. He and his work clothes reeked so bad that I was convinced that he was just getting paid for mixing and frying sugar and shit, glazing it, and selling it as doughnuts. That night, I thought the bed moving was him, but when I sniffed and didn't detect the DEFCON odor, I knew he wasn't home yet, and that I was alone. I assumed that the mattress shaking was nothing and happily closed my eyes into more funk-free sleep.

The bed shook again, and I looked to my right toward the bedroom door. My eyes opened to a pair of knees covered in chocolate-brown slacks. Don't ask me how I knew that the person was black skinned, had masculine energy, and wore a really nice eighties' television sitcom–style cable-knit sweater with patterned hues of beige, chestnut, and cocoa brown that matched his neatly pleated slacks. I didn't look up to see his face, but I intuitively knew that he was pointing over me toward the green wall behind me. I turned away from the pointing man to my left and faced the plain wall and saw nothing but rotating shadows and streetlights reflecting from the window fan, but I did hear a baby crying. The crying seemed to stop as soon as it started, and I was wide awake. Immediately, I turned back to my right, and the man standing at the foot of my bed was gone—just like that.

I wasn't new to visitors from the other side. I grew up in a family where feeling, seeing, and talking to Spirits was an everyday thing. My grandma said it came from being born with a veil over your face. Although we were practicing Catholics, five generations removed from Germany on my momma's side, talking with the dead beyond Mary and Jesus wasn't really viewed as double-timing Christ, especially if talking to the dead brought much needed "tea" from the other side: dreams of slithering snakes to let you know to watch out because someone you really trusted was going to betray you; regular warnings to ignore short and dark haints (ghosts) promising winning lottery numbers and other secret riches in exchange for your soul. My grandma's best girlfriend, who died young, regularly entered the world of the living through my grandma's south bedroom wall to forewarn Grandma first of her son's death and then later of her daughter's, my momma's, death. Uncle Freddie, my grandma's dead brother, who died in a car twisted around a sneaky bend on a southern Illinois back highway after too much whiskey, always confirmed Grandma's suspicions of Pawpaw's infidelity with that light-skinned hussy at the bar. And the old white lady, the former owner of my grandmother's nineteenth-century home, stomped nightly through the shotgun hallways and seemed to really get off on revealing herself, only her head, in full living color to folks who were courageous enough to sleep in her former bedroom and make the fatal error of looking up at the ceiling right before they fell asleep.

"Did you know who it was?" Grandma would ask me if I saw or sensed somebody when we spent our preteen summers with her.

"No," I responded.

"Well. They ain't gonna bother you if you don't bother them. Don't be scared. If you are scared, just ask them, 'What in the name of the Lord do you want?' and they should go away. It is the living that should scare you and not the dead," she always calmly replied.

About two years earlier, in 1998, I had lost a baby at six weeks. I had no pain or other symptoms, except for some spotting. If it weren't for a faint blue line on the Walgreens pregnancy test and the absence of a regular period, I wouldn't have known any difference in my body. In some ways, it was like it had never happened. I had just finished graduate school, and at the end of the summer, I realized that I had missed my period. I went to the doctor's office. My sister and I were the only black people in the waiting room of the clinic, and we seemed to wait forever. Finally, a nurse called me to the front desk of the clinic and asked me to go pee in a cup. I followed the nurse to the back, entered the bathroom, peed in the plastic cup after wiping from front to back with a moist towelette, and followed the nurse back into the public waiting room. The nurse told me and my sister to remain in the public waiting room for the test results. My sister and I kept looking at each other, wondering if we stunk or something, because we wondered why the nurse, a white woman, couldn't just allow us to wait in a patient room for the results.

Twenty years later I can see the dismissiveness and institutional racism in the nurse's action,[1] but back then I was so grateful to have completed my master's degree and to have made it that far in life. I think I was just doing enough just to make it through the situation, just enough to make it through every day. I hadn't planned on having a child then, but I naively and arrogantly believed at the time that I would be fine because I wasn't a teenager and I had completed my education. With the best of intentions, I had been so trained as a black girl growing up in poverty on the south side of Chicago not to get pregnant and to complete my education. Little did I know that my so-called success and *ed-u-ma-ca-tion* only increased my mortality risk and the likelihood that I would miscarry, and that I was more likely to die from complications from pregnancy and childbirth.[2] I wondered if my white doctors and nurses understood this fact and if they even cared.

Once the nurse returned with the results, it seemed that because I had not yet made it to the first trimester, I wasn't worthy of seeing a doctor and waiting in an actual patient room. Apparently, my human chorionic gonadotropin (hCG) levels were not high enough for the length of time that

I had been without a period, which was told to me and my sister in the public waiting room. We were not afforded the human dignity of privacy. I kept asking questions, and finally we were escorted to a waiting room, where a white female nurse did an ultrasound. It was confirmed that the fetus was dead, or in their words, "nonviable." The nurse also informed me that fetal loss in the first trimester is so normal that they, the medical establishment, don't even consider it an issue or problem unless a woman experiences three miscarriages in a row. It was all so very nonchalant and matter-of-fact that I felt like I maybe had overreacted. Maybe I did something wrong. The nurse explained that the uterus and body would naturally expel the fetus, including tissue, and if it did not expel from the body in a couple of weeks, I was to return to the doctor.

I felt like I was in a daze and that a cruel trick had been played on me. I had spent over sixteen years, since sixth grade, making sure that I didn't have a baby, that I didn't stink—as my sixth-grade teacher had warned us girls during "the talk" about our periods and wearing deodorant—and working hard to outlive my membership in the sixth-grade brown birds math group, as opposed to the red cardinals and blue jays math groups. Here, sixteen years later, in 1998, I had been responsible, I got *ed-u-macated*, fell in love, and now—finally—wanted to have a baby, and my body and the Universe were like "Fuck You!" The next week on Wednesday, which would have been the first day of my graduate writing program, I felt a quick tearing inside my belly and rushed to the bathroom. I missed my first class of the semester, a fiction class—the novel—and I spent that evening sitting long periods on the toilet with the steady sound of skin and blood clots dropping and flopping into water to keep me company. Even after all that, I was still in love with that skinny black guy named for Jesus, and I still wanted to have his babies.

Maybe my miscarriage was a punishment, and I wondered if black women could have it all: babies, education, a career, and love.

...

Before I became pregnant in 1998, my momma came to me in a dream, as she often did in the year after her sudden death in 1997 at the age of forty-nine. On one visit, she told me about men, "that God will choose." I had no clue what the hell she was talking about, but when my current love interest *at the time,* Sphincter Muscle, "Sphinc" or "Satan II" for short, started complaining of someone beating him in the head at night and waking him out of his sleep, I knew it was my momma. It was funny as hell to see how scared his community-dick-having-self was, but it still took me a couple of months to leave his trifling ass, because the sex was really good. From my late teens through my twenties, I had several relationships, had experienced my own loves, and watched the loves of family members disintegrate, and I knew and believed then, unequivocally, that I did not want to have any children.

"You will never find a husband and get married!" My grandma would yell at me when I, twelve years old and knowing it all, complained about my required daily chores of cleaning her house, which included the dreaded vacuum. My mother would send me and my older sister to stay with my grandma during the summers of the late eighties. I now realize it was another birth control strategy and to keep us away from what she feared could happen to latchkey kids in the summer streets of Chicago, latchkey black girls home alone. It's ironic to think that my mother and her mother, Grandma, actually believed that it was harder for two preteen black girls to get pregnant living in a small southern Illinois town in the middle of nowhere instead of on the south side of Chicago with too much time on your hands.

"I don't want to get married and have a husband!" I would yell back at my grandma when she chastised me for not wanting to be her maid and clean her house every day.

My grandma would just look at me and shake her head. She really believed that she was living the life, and from her viewpoint I guess it made sense. She was born and raised in the Great Depression, and I can't imagine how dangerous it must have been for a pretty black girl growing up in a small mining town run through by train tracks in southern Illinois in the 1930s and 1940s. As my grandma explained, she worked, cooked, took care of the kids, and cleaned the house, and my Pawpaw worked, paid the bills, fixed stuff around the house, kept the garden, and drank at the VFW every night. I do mean every night.

She and Pawpaw had five kids, and the oldest child, Mark Anthony, was stillborn. I knew this from as long as I could remember because my mother always talked about her stillborn brother, Mark. My momma so loved Mark that she named my baby brother, Ronnie, after him, but she ended up changing his name from Mark to my father's name, Ronald, because my father (Satan I) threw a stone-cold fit. Although my father had completely abandoned the family by the time that my baby brother was born, and even went so far as to tell people that my brother Ronnie wasn't his, my father still expected my mother to name her last and fifth child, my brother, after him and not her dead stillborn brother. I was only eight years old then, but I understood. I wanted Momma not to cave to my father, but she did. It was like my father believed he owned my momma, her uterus, and what came out of it, even when he treated her and us, his children, like shit.

I guess it was hard because when my brother, Ronnie, was born, he looked like my father literally spit him out. I guess my father was my first relationship with a Sphincter Muscle. I could not understand a world where a man could marry a woman, have five kids with her, and walk away from her and his own kids and lead a life as if those kids did not come out of his nut sac, as if their mother who carried them in her body for nine months and pushed them out of her vagina did not exist. Where they do that at? Now you know why I, initially, was not down for the baby thing. That shit is just jacked up, and I had (have) issues, and I was never going to make myself that vulnerable to another human being.

...

Having grown up the second oldest of five kids and raised by a single mother, I experienced one of the best forms of birth control that exist. I was a mother of three kids at the age of eight. There were three siblings born after me, and by age eight, I was cooking, cleaning, changing diapers, and babysitting my sisters and brother because my mother had to go to work during the day to provide for us. By this time, my father had completely abandoned the family. I could count on one hand how many times from age eight through eighteen that I actually saw my father in a year's time, and just because I saw him didn't mean that he recognized and acknowledged me or my siblings as his children in those moments.

As experienced by most single mothers, particularly women of color, our father's physical abandonment of the family instantly left us in poverty. Although my mother worked tirelessly to keep a roof over our heads, there were many days when we went without basic necessities like heat, water, electricity, and sufficient food. I lived those ten years after my father left the house bearing witness to my mother's simultaneous suffering and tenacity, as a result of my father's betrayal and her structural social position as a single black woman parent living in the urban North in the United States. I watched my mother's body become emaciated as she continually took the smallest piece of fried chicken at dinner to ensure that her five growing children had enough food. She wore coats and boots years beyond their physical utility in the bitter cold and windy Chicago winters because she spent what little money she had on warm clothes and boots for her growing kids. At night, she made us put on our winter coats and boots and squeeze in tight together on our only couch, and then she placed blankets over us in the hope that our small bodies would not freeze during the night in the below-zero winter weather, because our heat had been cut off for nonpayment. And when my period first started at the age of twelve, she screamed on a regular basis for my first year of bleeding, "You can get pregnant now!"—instead of the ideal *Pretty in Pink* Molly Ringwald black girl experience that I really wanted.[3]

Then, I believed and was resentful that I never had a chance to be a little girl or a teenager. Instead, while my mother was constantly making preemptive stealth moves and running rescue missions to ensure that her five babies lived beyond the womb despite the personal, historical, and social economic conditions that forced the contrary on the daily, I played mother and father to myself and to my baby brother and sisters.

There is one Christmas photo after my father left the family and my mother had given birth to my brother, Ronnie, the previous summer. My mother is wearing a white dress, and our backs are to the kitchen door because we don't have a tree or gifts for this Christmas. We have pretty dresses, we have a new baby brother, we don't have enough food, and we have love. I can't remember who took the photo, but I am 100 percent sure that it was not my father.

I have looked at the photo a million times over the years, and I always assumed that it was a happy time because for the most part, it was a happy memory for me. In the picture, my sisters and I are smiling black girls, not recognizing or understanding at the time our momma's pain, suffering, strength, and sacrifice. It would be later after my mother's death in 1997 that my momma's mother, my grandma, would let a big-ass bone fall out of her mouth to tell us that my younger and only brother, Ronnie, had been a twin. That while pregnant and going through the stress of my father's infidelity, abandonment, and financial struggles, my momma miscarried my baby brother's brother.

It was not until I had my own children that I looked at the photo again and could see how emaciated and tired my momma really was, while my sisters and I stood in front of her body, taking from it. That in its stance, although weary, her body was an unwavering foundation of our full black girls' beauty and happiness of what all we knew, even in our poverty, as we wore our beautifully white detailed frilly dresses that Momma had sewn by hand, every stitch filled with the best of love, devotion, courage, and strength that she could give us.

53

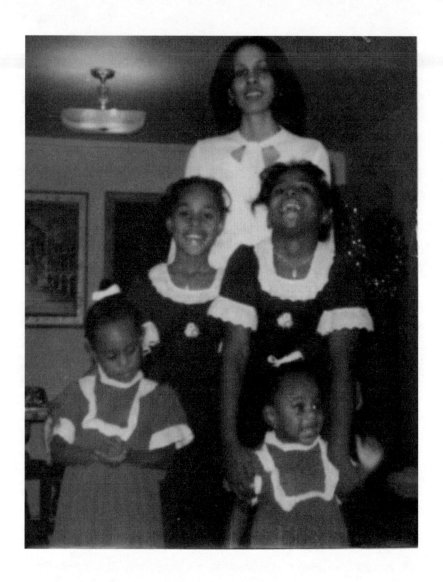

...

"Don't you ever let a man do to you what your father did to me," my mother would preach to us daily until I left home for college at the age of seventeen, and you best believe that by high school, I had Planned Parenthood on speed dial, and I knew the quickest CTA bus route to the nearest clinic. Although I didn't fully understand it then, my mother was trying to tell me in her own way and in the words that she understood that my ability to have agency and control over my uterus, my choice to procreate, and my mental, emotional, and physical health would directly connect to my ability to access my dreams, autonomy, liberty, citizenship, and equity as a black woman living in this world.

I have a tilted, retroverted uterus. Although a uterus can become tilted for many reasons, some women are born with a tipped uterus. From my first pap smear as a teenager, once doctors discovered that my uterus was retroverted, they treated me like a specimen in a cage. With permission of course, OB-GYNs would call in their colleagues and students for an opportunity to *see* my uterus, live and direct, shifted back as a result of heredity. My young sister, the third child, has a bicornuate, or heart-shaped, uterus, and she successfully carried and birthed two healthy children. Having a heart-shaped uterus is genetic, too. Like a preening large cat, I used to think that my uterus was special, until I learned that one out of every five women has a tilted uterus, and it is really a fairly common physical condition.

In the essay "Crooked Room" from *Sister Citizen: Shame, Stereotypes, and black Women America*, Dr. Harris-Perry notes that "black women are standing in a crooked room, and they have to figure out which way is up. Bombarded with warped images of their humanity, some black women tilt and bend themselves to fit the distortion" (29). She goes on to argue that despite the public and political actions of black women that may contradict stereotypes, the reality is that "it can be hard to stand up straight in a crooked room" (29).[4]

Maybe God tilted my uterus because S/HE understood the social economic challenges and contradictions that I would face as a black woman
born into this crooked world that makes it hard for black and brown
women to stand straight, to find equilibrium. My uterus's slight tilt, like
the universal black greeting of the head nod with an explicit or implicit
"What's up?"[5] allowed me the ability to find equilibrium despite the constant distortions caused by the intersectionality of gendered, racial, and
class oppression that I and my body, my uterus, and my dead, born, and
unborn black babies have experienced. The tilt in my uterus might be the
only physical thing keeping me and other women, especially brown and
black women, upright.

A year after I left "Sphinc, i.e., Satan II" in 1998, I met a black skinny man
who told me that his name, Emmanuel, means that "God is with Us." All
I could think about was that he had the prettiest set of white teeth and
the kindest brown eyes that I had ever seen. He was the gentlest person
that I had ever met. Emmanuel explained that he initially wanted to be a
priest, so he was right with God. When he smiled at me for the first time
and asked if he could carry my book bag back to my apartment, I really
knew that Jesus was indeed with us, as my ovaries actually tingled for real
for real, and I knew that I was in trouble. All my years of shit-talking about
wanting to have absolutely no kids went out the front door. Three months
later, after meeting a black man with a name that meant "Jesus is with us,"
I was pregnant at age twenty-eight, overeducated, unmarried, unem-
ployed, in love, full of hope, and so excited to have a baby. For the first
time in my life, I felt free, and that I could do anything that I wanted.

That August summer night in 2000 in the Iowa suburb, I didn't recognize
the black man in the brown slacks and sweater that stood by and shook
my bed while I slept. I jumped up, turned on the lights, and went to the
bathroom. In my family, Spirits only came to visit to bring messages, pri-
marily death. I couldn't go back to sleep, and waited for Emmanuel to

arrive from work. After making sure that he had showered and placed his uniform and shoes in a hermetically sealed plastic trash bag left outside the bedroom, I allowed him to enter the room. With a great deal of hubris, I suggested to Emmanuel that he phone home to make sure that everyone was all right, because I believed that I recognized every Spirit that had ever approached me. Since I didn't recognize the black man in brown pants, it must have been a visit for Emmanuel.

Although I had been cramping in my lower abdomen over the past week and my OB-GYN had diagnosed me with uterine fibroids, telling me that women carried full healthy babies to term perfectly with uterine fibroids, it wasn't in the realm of my imagination to even consider that my almost five-month-old baby in my stomach could die—again.

The next morning Emmanuel and I woke to start our drive to Minnesota, as we were moving there, and I was headed back to graduate school to complete my program. That morning I had been experiencing painful cramping without any blood, and I called my OB-GYN clinic. I thought maybe that I should go to the emergency room, but neither I nor Emmanuel had any health insurance at the time.

I left an urgent message for the doctor.

He called me back.

"You can go to the emergency room, but they are only going to give you Tylenol and send you home. Just take Tylenol, and you will be fine," he said matter-of-factly.

Although in great pain, I trusted the doctor and didn't go to the emergency room. I took Tylenol, and Emmanuel and I set out that day for our three- to four-hour drive to Minneapolis.

An hour south of the Minnesota border on Interstate 35, I felt a pop, and water gushed down my legs and pooled at my sandal-covered feet.

I could hear myself screaming, "No! No! No! No!" thinking that if I said it loud enough it could stop the water from running out of my body.

Emmanuel pulled to the side of the road, and we decided that we would drive to the nearest hospital.

When we arrived at the hospital, I told them that my water had broken.

I remember sitting in a wheelchair in the hallway as people walked past me like they did not want to touch me. People walked past me like they did not see me.

I sat there in the wheelchair thinking that as long as I didn't stand up, water would not flow out of my uterus.

All the people in the hospital were white.

I just kept praying that the water, the amniotic fluid, remained in my womb.

When I finally was given a room while they asked for information about my OB-GYN, they called my doctor and waited for his response. I lay in the hospital bed and cried while Emmanuel held my hand. The nurses kept asking for the name of my primary physician, but I only had an OB-GYN.

As I write this essay, I realize that I was college educated, twenty-eight years old, and I didn't have a primary doctor. I didn't see a doctor regularly or yearly unless there was something wrong. I didn't go to the doctor unless I had to. Going to the doctor was never an enjoyable or comfortable experience for me as a woman of color, and the one moment when I really needed a doctor, it felt like I didn't have one, because the OB-GYN seemed to just be going through the motions. The OB-GYN made me feel like he didn't care about me. I wondered if the OB-GYN was married, and if his wife was pregnant with fibroids and cramping would he have told her to take Tylenol, or would he have insisted that she go to the emergency room.

I don't remember much about the exam in the emergency room, but doctors were in agreement that my water had broken; however, I was not going into labor as they expected. It was then that I finally realized that my stomach cramping had stopped.

A doctor from my clinic, not my OB-GYN from that same clinic, finally called the emergency room, and he, with a kind voice, advised me to return and be admitted to the hospital where the clinic was located to see if the amniotic fluid would fill back up in the sac. The doctor said that sometimes the fluid builds back up in the amniotic sac. I was hopeful, and Emmanuel and I returned to the hospital near the clinic, and I was admitted.

I was in the hospital for seven days. During those days I can only remember feeling the baby move and me crying. It was my first time to feel the baby move because I was close to twenty weeks. The doctor told me that I could feel the baby move because there was no longer any fluid in the amniotic sac. I was constantly worried that the baby was feeling pain and could not breathe properly because there was so much fluid loss. After a week, the hospital doctors realized that my amniotic sac was not going to refill with amniotic fluid, so they gave me the option of inducing labor or a D&C. After feeling the baby for that entire week, I couldn't imagine them doing a D&C on the baby, so we opted for induction. It was then, after a week of crying, waiting, and drinking as much water as one could imagine, that I realized that my original OB-GYN doctor from the clinic never visited me in the hospital. He never came to the hospital room, and he never even called.

It was then that doctor, a different OB-GYN than my OB-GYN at the clinic, told me that all the time I had been cramping and experiencing what I felt was like really bad period cramps and the baby just growing, I was really in labor. I didn't know it because I had never given birth to a baby, and my clinic OB-GYN did not inform me of this. My uterine fibroids were intramural, submucosal, and subserosal. In other words, the tumors were inside my uterus, embedded into the walls of my uterus, and on the outside walls of my uterus, and they put pressure on the amniotic sac until it burst because there wasn't enough room inside my uterus for both the growing fibroids and the growing baby from where the placenta was attached.[6]

Because of my uterine fibroids, I should have been classified as a high-risk pregnancy, and when I called the clinic doctor the night before we left for our trip to Minnesota complaining of really bad cramping, the clinic doctor should have told me to go to the nearest emergency room immediately in order to try to stop my labor, as I was automatically high risk for miscarriage since I had fibroids. You can do everything you are supposed to do, and stuff can still go left.

I was placed in a labor-and-delivery room. The room seemed really empty as there were no extra accessories: no infant bed with a warmer, no baby blankets, no bassinet, so scale, no fetal monitors, no maternity kits, etc. This was a room for a dead baby with the barest of essentials, as the doctor had told us that the baby would not survive the birth. Even then, I was still hoping.

I naively believed that the labor would not be difficult, because I rationalized that the baby was so small. What damage could an almost twenty-week fetus do to the body?

I was given a morphine drip and a Pitocin drip. At first it wasn't that bad, but I quickly reached my maximum drug allowance on the morphine, and it started to hurt really badly.

"It hurts, it hurts, it hurts . . ." were the only words I had for Emmanuel.

It was like it was not happening to me, and I was floating above the room just watching it and recording it in my memory for future recall. Like a person under duress, I knew my job was just to merely get through it. I was used to the worst things happening and knowing how to survive and appear normal in spite of them.

"Can you press again? It really hurts," I asked Emmanuel.

"You've reached your maximum dose," he told me.

Once I was fully dilated, the baby came, and she was a girl.

"I can see her chest moving! See! She's breathing! She's breathing!" I told the doctor as he held her, and I watched him gently come over to me and press his thumb over her chest reminding me that she was too small for any instruments to aid her. I think I thought if I looked at her hard enough and concentrated that she would come back to life.

She was so tiny and beautiful. I just kept smelling her because she smelled so good and so different. I had never smelled anything like it. She smelled like something from another world, and it smelled so good. My baby did not stink, and I couldn't believe that she came out of me and that I smelled that good on the inside. Even in that moment I wondered why my sixth-grade teacher had taught us that black girls stink. I knew then that she was a liar. Since my baby came out of me smelling so good, then I must be good, too. I just wanted her to be good with me and to stay with me. I think I kept her blankets for over ten years, just to take them out of their special box to smell them every now and then.

We called the priest to give last rites, and when he entered the room, we showed him our baby, who to us was the most beautiful girl in the world. The white Catholic priest physically recoiled as if he had seen something repulsive. I thought, "I'm Catholic, and Emmanuel is Catholic, named after Jesus. Why wouldn't he want to baptize our baby girl and give her last rites?"

The hardest was leaving the hospital and leaving her there. I kept wanting to go back and to look and touch her body, and I did. I knew it was not healthy, but I just wanted to keep looking at her and touching her just one more time. I couldn't stop myself. We took pictures, but I kept feeling like I would forget her, and it is the worst feeling in the world to believe that you are going to forget what your child looks like because you know that you won't see her face again. We finally decided to have her cremated because as students we were not attached to any place, and I could not imagine burying her in a place where we didn't live and then she would be there alone and all by herself. Our daughter was cremated and placed in a brass urn, which I still have placed on an altar today with pictures of my mother, grandmothers, auntie, and uncle, all of whom have passed.

Sylvia Browne, a prominent psychic, was scheduled to come to the Twin Cities in 2001,[7] and unbeknownst to Emmanuel, I splurged and bought tickets for us to see her. Pregnant again, I was about twenty weeks along, and we were living in an apartment in south Minneapolis. We were both working and in school. The arena where Sylvia Browne was speaking was full to capacity, and Emmanuel and I were seated on the main floor in the back. By this time, we had been together for over two years, and he was used to my fascination with Spirits. Plus, he was named after Jesus, so how could he not be as well?

That night Sylvia Browne held a lottery for all ticket holders to choose what lucky ones would go to the stage to ask her a question directly. I was not one of the lucky ones. I had two chances because Emmanuel told me that he would have given me his ticket if his number was called. I told ya'll he was sweet. Anyway, Browne led the entire auditorium through a guided meditation, and she advised everyone to individually ask in their heads the question that we would like our Higher Power, in my case God/Universe, to answer for us.

"Will my baby make it past twenty-five weeks?"

"Will my baby make it past twenty-five weeks?"

"Please God, will my baby make it past twenty-five weeks?" I kept asking this question over and over again in my head like a mantra, a prayer. Although these questions were a part of my guided meditation with Sylvia Browne in that moment in the auditorium there in St. Paul sitting next to Emmanuel, this question had been my obsession since we found out that we were pregnant again.

"You call us anytime for any concerns that you have about your pregnancy. It's better to be safe than sorry, and our job is to make you feel at ease," is what the clinic nurse in 2001 told me.

This time, we had an OB-GYN who diagnosed me as a high-risk pregnancy, and I received the additional and needed medical care, compassion, and concern relative to my medical condition and risks.[8] My OB-GYN was part of a clinic that specifically served women of color and understood the unique risks and disparities relative to women of color and pregnancy: hypertensive disorders, diabetes, fibroids, education, and poverty.[9] They made me feel like they cared, and they listened to me and responded to my questions and needs. I knew that there were never any guarantees, but Emmanuel and I felt confident in our health care and pregnancy this time around. We felt that we were receiving care from experts who met our medical needs and actually cared about the success of our pregnancy, birth, and child.

...

The guided mediation with Sylvia Browne ended, I felt refreshed, and Emmanuel and I drove back to our basement apartment in south Minneapolis.

That night, I was awakened by someone shaking the bed. We had graduated to a full bed, and I was lying flat on my back, and my right side was on the edge. I looked to my right, and there was the same black man with the brown pants and sweater that I first saw in the summer of 2000. He had returned, but this time he was not alone. There was someone standing next to him to his right, dressed in a glowing white robe like a Roman toga.

Again, I seemed not to lift my eyes high enough to see their faces. The person in the white robe had an open book in his hand, and he lifted his right hand and pointed directly to my stomach while the black man in brown looked at the man in white. The black man in brown then jumped into my stomach, and my whole body shook and vibrated from my tummy throughout my entire frame, and a feeling of complete peace and knowingness fell over me. I knew then that I had watched my child's soul enter her body and that the baby I was carrying, right then and there in 2001, was going to be all right.

I looked to my left, and saw that Emmanuel, Jesus, had slept through the entire thing. I realized in that moment that back when my bed shook during that hot, muggy August night in 2000, my daughter's Spirit had come to tell me, "Mommy, not yet." She was letting me know that it wasn't her time but trying to explain to me that she would return, and on that night in 2001 her soul did just that.

As bad-ass as I pretended to and wanted to be, I decided that I couldn't be a fifth-generation *recovering* Catholic with a Catholic baby daddy named Jesus and not get married. With an eight-month-full belly, Emmanuel and I were married at the Hennepin County Courthouse. My baby brother, Ronnie, and my sister with the heart-shaped uterus stood as witnesses.

Our daughter was born thirty-three days later at nine pounds and twenty-one inches long. I prayed during my twelve hours and seventeen minutes of labor that I would see my mother, but I didn't, and I named my daughter after her anyway.

Notes

1 See P. R. Lockhart, "What Serena Williams's Scary Childbirth Story Says about Medical Treatment of Black Women: Black Women Are Often Dismissed or Ignored by Medical Care Providers. Williams Wasn't an Exception," vox.com, January 11, 2018, https://www.vox.com/identities/2018/1/11/16879984/serena-williams-childbirth-scare-black-women.

2 According to Reeves and Matthew, "The infant mortality rate for black babies is twice that for whites. But this is not a poverty story. Babies born to well educated, middle-class black mothers are more likely to die before their first birthday than babies born to poor white mothers with less than a high school education." See Richard V. Reeves and Dayna Bowen Matthew, "Social Mobility Memos: Six Charts Showing Race Gaps within the American Middle Class," Brookings.com, October 21, 2016, https://www.brookings.edu/blog/social-mobility-memos/2016/10/21/6-charts-showing-race-gaps-within-the-american-middle-class/. Also see K. C. Schoendorf and C. J. R. Hogue, "Mortality among Infants of Black as Compared with White College-Educated Parents," *New England Journal of Medicine* 326, no. 23 (1992): 1522–27, EBSCO host.

3 *Pretty in Pink,* directed by Howard Deutch, with Molly Ringwald, Jon Cryer, and Harry Dean Stanton (Paramount Pictures, 1986).

4 Melissa Harris-Perry, "Crooked Room," in *Sister Citizen: Shame, Stereotypes, and Black Women in America, for Colored Girls Who've Considered Politics When Being Strong Isn't Enough* (New Haven, Conn.: Yale University Press, 2011), 28–50.

5 Musa Okwonga, "The Nod: A Subtle Lowering of the Head You Give to Another Black Person in an Overwhelmingly White Place," Medium, October 16, 2014, https://medium.com/matter/the-nod-a-subtle-lowering-of-the-head-to

-another-black-person-in-an-overwhelmingly-white-place-e12bfa0f833f.

6 According to Elizabeth A. Stewart and colleagues, "Multiple lines of evidence suggest that uterine fibroids have a disproportional effect on African-American women. African-American women have a higher cumulative risk of uterine fibroids, a threefold greater incidence and relative risk of fibroids, and an earlier age of onset. In addition, African-American women are 2.4 times more likely to undergo hysterectomy and have a 6.8-fold increase of undergoing uterine-sparing myomectomy. At the time of hysterectomy, African-American women have higher uterine weights, more fibroids, a higher likelihood of preoperative anemia, and more severe pelvic pain. Data also suggests that African-American women may have biologically distinct disease." Elizabeth A. Stewart, Wanda K. Nicholson, Linda Bradley, and Bijan J. Borah, "The Burden of Uterine Fibroids for African-American Women: Results of a National Survey," *Journal of Women's Health* 22, no. 10 (2013): 807–16, PMC.

7 Sylvia Browne (1936–2013) was a psychic, medium, author, and spiritual teacher.

8 Kiera Butler, "A Surprisingly Simple Way Black Women Can Reduce Pregnancy Risks," MotherJones.com, July/August 2018, https://www.motherjones.com/politics/2018/08/simple-way-reduce-risk-black-pregnancy-premature-birth/.

9 Linda Villarosa, "Why America's Black Mothers and Babies Are in a Life-or-Death Crisis: The Answer to the Disparity in Death Rates Has Everything to Do with the Lived Experience of Being a Black Woman in America," *New York Times Magazine,* April 11, 2018, https://www.nytimes.com/2018/04/11/magazine/black-mothers-babies-death-maternal-mortality.html.

The Pursuit of Happiness

Jennifer N. Baker

It ends as quickly as it began. The latest cramp a punch in the gut. You convulse in bed and go fetal from impact. The moisture in your underwear spreads, and it's as though you pissed yourself. This liquid is thicker though, pungent in a different way, not of ammonia but acrid. You turn away from the full-length mirror reflecting the mattress. You're glad for the evening, for the shadows and lack of moonlight filtering in from the bedroom window creating slivers of ivory along the floor. You don't want to see your face when another rumble hits your abdomen.

* * *

A week earlier you watched as your sisters-in-law bustled around Mrs. Smith, who stood like a general commandeering her squad in the kitchen. "There's something about a woman in heels with a string of pearls," Joel said, "that makes you know she means business." The women fulfilled the prerequisite duties for dinner of plating, divvying up cutlery, tasting items that you all had no real say in but knew by now to adjust your expectations and your taste buds.

The husbands shuffled in and out, familiar with their part in this performance. They asked if they could help, were shooed away with a playful flick of a hand towel as they dipped a finger in sauce or picked at a chicken thigh, before shuffling off not to be seen again in this space. You stood waiting by the door frame, offering yourself. You were in that in-between place: not stranger, not family. You knew more acutely in that moment this would change.

"You sit and relax, Mikayla," Mrs. Smith said, not giving you the kindness of a swat or a gesture of mock annoyance. She was polite in a way that read as anything but, though she was practiced enough to know the difference, and you'd been with Joel long enough to see it as well.

Once everyone was seated in the dining room, grace recited by Dr. Smith in the form of "Rub a dub dub thanks for the grub," followed by an eye roll from Mrs. Smith, you announced, "I'm pregnant." You said this for the second time in a year to your in-laws. Once again it was received with cheers that punctuated off the wineglasses, echoing in the usually quiet space.

Dr. Smith, big, imposing, an aged linebacker—he continues to urge you to call him William—was the first to get up from his place at the head to hug you. He held your face with hands that felt like slabs on your cheeks. "Our first one." His eyes were intense, not the ice blue of Joel and his mother and brothers but hard and dark.

"Calls for a drink," Mike said, downing his in one gulp and already making his way to the crystal bottles against the wall.

Mrs. Smith was next. "Congratulations, dear." She smiled. It wasn't slight either. Her lips etched parentheses into her cheeks.

She was gentle in that moment, a fragile-looking woman who was anything but. She reached out to squeeze your hand, you squeezed hers back, hoping this could be the white flag, so to speak. Tension had been apparent from the first day you set foot in the space she raised Joel and his brothers. You kept wondering if she disliked you because you were you, because you were black, or because you were not good enough for her son. Joel insisted none of the above was true. His mother had been this way his whole life.

Celebration continued after dinner. Mike had certainly lost count of how many drinks he'd had, though no one else did. The men stood clustered around the bar. The women huddled on love seats and cushioned chairs, in a room with ceramic vases and walls lined with framed degrees. Accomplishments served as decor.

"We're going to have to start thinking about the nursery," she said, encircling you into the "hen party," as she called it, consisting of you, Mrs. Smith, and Joel's brothers' wives. Now you were immersed in this world. Just like with the women at work. The ones who had families and once you said, "I'm pregnant," that partition blew apart, a drawbridge was lowered, and you were allowed into the fold because motherhood? That transcends everything.

From your new membership location, you watched your husband get commended. Noticed Jerry stare at you before catching your gaze and looking away. You saw Joel smile, and his cheeks reddened, almost eliminating the freckles lining his face when Mike said, "You and Mikayla have been busy, busy, busy." In that moment you saw why your sister commented your husband could give Shaun and David Cassidy a run for their money if performance was in his blood rather than medicine. Joel's face was childlike, sweet, and kind all at the same time. His slim frame and height gave him an advantage over most, but seeing a hand rub the back of his neck, that "aw shucks" Opie-type demeanor, you wanted to embrace him.

"Mikayla?" Mrs. Smith said, bringing your attention back to what you had missed. She cupped your chin, patted your cheek. Her fingers were cold. She examined you from head to toe with a glare only a mother knew how to use.

"You know," she began as if starting a story, "when I met you, you were a student, and then you weren't. Then you were a hostess, and then you weren't." Her lids lowered, shading her gaze slightly. "Then you were a secretary, and then you weren't."

You tensed and crossed your legs, waiting for her to pounce, expecting her to go through each position. You had edited your résumé enough times, had rubbed out and retyped over dates and responsibilities. Cursed at the holes in the paper wearing thin from all the erasures and having to start over. Your stomach curdled at the thought of the search, of finding a place to fit.

"But, perhaps," Mrs. Smith continued, "you found what you were looking for?" Her palm landed on the still-forming mound. Maybe she could feel something small inside there that Joel said he hadn't felt when you'd asked him earlier in the day.

"I don't care what any 'feminist' says," and here she leaned in as though sharing a secret between the two of you. "There is nothing wrong with wanting to be a mother and having a family, now is there?"

"N-n-no." Your voice came out more garbled than you had intended or wanted. "There isn't."

"You have something there let me get that," your mother-in-law insisted, quickly wiping away your tears before anyone else noticed.

"What are you thinking of for colors? You can go neutral or wait until you know the sex." The other wives remained quiet.

"I want to know. But I don't necessarily want an all-blue or all-pink room," you said, thinking more on it. Grinning as the words came out because it was happening. You'd be a mother. A role designated by you.

From across a room, genders and generations divided like a high school dance, you and your husband caught each other's eyes and you mouthed, "I'm happy."

* * *

You stay in bed for several minutes, hoping it's a fluke this time, that it's spotting and not a steady flow. The patch of reddish brown seeps into the sheets and spreads. It's then that you shed your clothing.

In the dark you maneuver out of the bedroom and into the bathroom next door. You almost fall into the toilet because the seat was left up. Your bones mash against porcelain, your butt slaps against cold water.

Slamming the lid, you take a seat and unclench your legs. You hunch your back, steel yourself waiting for the latest spasm to pass. Your body shudders from the pain, the feel of your uterus being twisted, waiting for this fetus to expel itself.

This is the third fetus gone, the second miscarriage with Joel. The first was six years ago, an abortion in 1975. As a tremor ripples from your belly button to your pelvis, you wonder if the warnings and admonishments were true. If that procedure, still experimental to legitimate practitioners several years ago, has screwed you for life. Or if the physician you trusted, the gung-ho man who touted *Roe v. Wade* like a theme song to inpatients, wasn't as knowledgeable as he claimed. You walked into the clinic, into the medicinal smell of a place where procedures were done. When you placed your feet in stirrups, you weren't nervous, you were anxious. Anxious to remove something that would tie you to a partner you did not love, something that could deter you from the destiny your mother held on to since your youth. Medical school was months away, and, as you believed at the time, the child growing inside of you was going to hinder that. After, there was discomfort, but it didn't extend beyond the physical. You didn't feel loss so much, but a reprieve. Funny how things change.

If you weren't already wincing from the cramps, you'd smack yourself for announcing this pregnancy. You're only six weeks gone this time, before you were four when you lost it.

You knew better. Beyond the confirmation from urinating in a cup and later on a stick, there was nothing. No nausea, no yeast infection, no hormonal imbalance that you could speak of. And the pain? The pulsing in your crotch is just what you deserve.

* * *

"I'm pregnant," you said to a different family a few days prior. There was less fanfare than with the Smiths.

Your mother and sister stopped their respective chopping and peeling in the kitchen. Your father was in his La-Z-Boy with Joel beside him on the couch. They'd been in conversation over their unifier: baseball. Your husband and father were animated, the wood paneling on the wall behind them served as a backdrop like they were on Dick Cavett or something. Wilhemina's husband and your brother were elsewhere in the house or neighborhood, oh but they'd be around once the food was ready.

The buffer between the kitchen the ladies prepped in and the living room the men sat in was a thin wall with a hole. A counter erect between the rooms reminded you of the times you and your brothers got on chairs and pretended your mother was your own private waitress. "My life is not to serve," she'd say. You all gaped at her with faces that'd been gob-smacked that a parent wasn't there for their child and their child alone.

Your father clapped Joel on the back, a universal congratulation among men, and said he was happy for you both. The cheeks you inherited glazed and rose as your father approached to kiss you on them. His scent of tonic and lacquer enveloped you when he embraced you.

"Sunday dinner isn't going to make itself," your mother said, and so everyone took their places again. You claimed your spot in the kitchen.

There was silence, or as silent as it could be with a toddler roaming around and announcers on the television shouting plays and stats. Music played dully on the ham radio your mother kept in the kitchen, splattered in grease and everything else that popped and sputtered from the stovetop.

Cutting cheese blocks into slices, you peeked at your sister's body, at the pouches that had yet to go away. You took note of motherhood lining Wilhemina's face, how it racked her figure. You already felt it, the flesh pushing itself out, being inflated, the swells. All of the blood pumping through you to your child.

You popped a chunk of Muenster in your mouth before putting the block back in the freezer. "Mmm, that's the good stuff," you said mid-chew, queueing your sister to respond, "Not as good as government cheese though." Wilhemina leaned back in her chair so she could see Joel in the adjoining room. "Right, Joel?"

"Leave the man alone," your father called, attempting to hide a laugh. When Joel was first introduced to your family, government cheese had been mentioned offhand, and he asked, "What's government cheese?" to stares from every Jenkins in the room. None of you had ever needed it, but you all knew what it was. "You've got cute going for you, that's for sure," your sister had told Joel.

"Yeah, leave my husband alone," you echoed. In the doorway you winked at your chided partner. "You want me to take her down? 'Cause I will if I have to." You flexed an arm.

Joel smiled at the television. "Remember, nonviolent resistance, M. I believe in healing, not fighting."

"And it's what I love about you. Among other things."

"I'd like a list of things you love about me at some point."

Your father lifted a hand in the air, his way of shushing. "I'm glad you love each other, but Randy is on the mound and our team is down."

"Little Randy Jackson plays baseball?" you asked only to receive a sigh from your father in return.

"Please don't joke with a man when his team is losing," your husband said, already putting a hand on your father's shoulder.

"Two runs! That's all we need."

Joel turned on his soothing tone, "I'm confident. There are two more innings left."

You wove around the women in a kitchen that was big for one yet small for three, nevertheless you made do because everyone had their area. Wilhemina at the rounded table for desserts and readying. Your mother at the counter. You on the farther counter next to the oven. Flowered wallpaper curled in on itself around the stove. The smells of onions and paprika, of cheddar and butter on noodles. The mustard greens and vinegar taking you home, further filling you up. You took another bite of Muenster warming in your hand.

"Are you eating all the cheese?" your mother asked, her voice on the cusp of scolding.

You offered a brazen grin with the evidence mashed on your tongue. "No."

Your mother's hands were slick with grease. She wiped them on the towel wedged between her torso and apron cinching all things culinary to her person. Her face was usually tight, but she was twitchy, blackheads dancing all over.

"What's up, Ma?" You approached her, slowly. "You're not happy for me?" you asked and gave her a quick squeeze from behind, smelling pepper on her inciting an itch through your nostrils in preparation for a sneeze.

She shrugged you off. Lifted an elbow to get you to step back because she was busy, and armed. "You're happy? I'm happy." It's what Joel said. "Are you happy about the baby?" "Sure. Whatever makes you happy makes me happy." It wasn't an answer and you told him so.

You recall the times as a child running into your mother and clutching her leg. Her patting your head and saying, "Alright now. I got work to do." Then you sprinting off elsewhere. There'll be no reassurances from your mother today.

You could almost feel your child push into your body until someone did in the form of your nephew. Sweet, honey-colored, and teething, he already had your skirt in his mouth. You hugged him and he smelled how a child should smell, sweet and sour with a touch of ointment. His cheeks are ripe like yours and your father's. He buried his head into you, more plush on plush. You breathed him in some more.

"He's not perfume, Mika," your sister said along with, "Try smelling him when his diaper's full."

His head was a warm stone that dribbled and drooled, still it was cute. "From afar," your sister tentatively agreed. You've seen her though. Witnessed her melting in the presence of her own children. But her softness is something she doesn't expose, even then her jaw was as tight as a man's, she blew the tendrils from her face and focused on her task, but her son smiled at her muttering "mama" and there it went, the edges shaved a bit at the acknowledgment of the voice saying it.

You kissed your nephew's head. "I was thinking I'd give notice in March. Mrs. Smith is urging me to quit, so is Joel, but I want to stay. The editor I work for likes me and, honestly, she scares me."

Your mother nodded but not in the way that denotes listening. Usually that was accompanied by a nod *and* the shifting of her body. At that moment she was ramrod, the stillness legendary as you kept speaking, hoping her hands would do something beyond working. That she'd say, "I'm happy for you," and mean it because ever since the dream she thought you and she shared was deferred on your side . . .

"I'll need help with some of the baby things. I haven't crocheted in a while so maybe we can get some needles and you can show me again."

Taking tiny hands in yours and guiding them. Teaching something to someone beyond how to xerox, fax, or make proper editing marks on a pile of manuscripts. The moments when your father guided you in driving or your mother supervised you chop and slice and grate were small, simple things that gave you an alternative perspective. Not of two parents telling, but showing. Wanting to make you a full-fledged person who *knew* things.

"We'll see," your mother said.

All it took was a moment, with Joel beside you and the words "I've quit" exiting your mouth that your mother morphed. She was "removed," no longer the thick arms that waddled in greeting wrapping around you to let you know you were home and you were good.

"It won't take long. I'm sure I'll remember again. Not sure why I—" you halted, not saying the word. Not laying gas to the grill, as your father would say, in terms of what you "gave up" once Joel came around.

"I like work, but that convention going on at Madison Square Garden is a pain," you said turning away from your mother. Chiding yourself for having a fleeting moment of being that same child who flung herself to legs waiting for the pat of acknowledgment.

"I can imagine," Wilhemina said. "Don't know why you don't work here."

"Pay's better."

"You don't even need the money." Your sister often slipped this into conversation.

"Well, I like it. Sometimes. Bigger. Different. More to see in the city. Art on the streets nowadays. Once the baby comes—"

Your mother intercepted, finally, "Mika, you may not want to start planning a whole future just yet."

"Why not?"

Your mother kept at the chicken, removing bone as quick as she deshelled beans. All of it fast movements, a deftness of her fingers from completing these tasks since childhood.

"Why not?" you pushed, but she still didn't reply. Fear, that's what it was. Creeping in, prickling in your extremities. Like she knew something you didn't. Like she could foresee the worst parts. Some high priestess ready with news but unwilling to spill it. "Ma?"

"I don't want you getting hurt."

Hurt? It was back to this then. "Joel isn't going to hurt me," you said.

That's when she looked at you, all knowing in her matriarchy. "Didn't say anything about Joel."

* * *

Your head is bent between your legs. Joel's mentioned this is the way to subdue dizziness. After an indeterminate amount of time, your limbs tingle from the numbness settling in. Rubbing your calves together there's the feel of stubble. Your feet are brown and shrunken, not gleaming and swollen like before. Then again, you may have imagined that.

Blood has gotten into the grout of the tile, missing the bathroom mat you squish under your toes. A brick-colored line runs through the beige.

Your home is your father-in-law's doing, the decor your mother-in-law's. Mrs. Smith encouraged clean lines, light colors.

The slam of the front door makes you sit up. Heat rushes to your head.

He shuffles rather than walks in the hallway. Joel's shoes scuff the floor.

He's close now. He hums to himself sometimes. Often to let you know he's on his way. The slight purr of Joel enough to alert you of his presence before the bed dips from his weight. You hear him on the way to the bedroom. The silence is what you wait for. The pause. He'll see the panties next to the bed, the sheets and comforter—a shame to mess up the silk you received as a wedding gift. Joel will see—

"Mikayla!"

You say nothing. No need to rush what will happen. Banging against the door. Joel calling frantically from the other side. The jiggle of the knob as he pushes into it. Damn thing is stuck. He bursts in, his face pink and sweaty. His scrubs and hair stick to his skin. His eyes are large and wondering. Joel fills the frame from top to bottom.

He switches on the light before crouching in front of you. You cover your eyes. Your vision strains adjusting to the brightness. The shade was sort of soothing. His knee covers the crevice of blood. Before you can tell him this, he paws you all over, warm fingers on cooling skin. Joel smells of musk but the room is all iron.

"How much blood have you lost?" he asks. He touches your forehead with the back of his hand, presses his index and middle fingers to your carotid artery. "Do you feel lightheaded?"

"No," you whisper.

"We should get you to the hospital." He grabs a towel from the rack behind him to cover your legs.

This is what reminds you why you couldn't be a doctor. How could you look at someone like yourself and summon up anything but pity? You imagine the women in this situation, those who experienced loss turning fragile, mute. Before quitting medical school, you saw these misfortunes firsthand and shrank away from them, instead becoming a doctor's wife. You'd be immobile as you are now, unable to step into action. Apologies would be the first thing to come to mind along with the immediate sensation to commiserate. This is what makes Joel a good doctor, his ability to focus, but at this moment you don't need a doctor.

"I'm not lightheaded."

"We should make sure. I'll call ahead—"

Whatever look you send cuts him off. You repeat his name. He gives you a once-over. Those eyes reading you the way he has since you first met. This is a time for comfort.

Joel rubs your knuckles with his thumb. "I'm sorry," he says. "I'm so, so sorry. I know how much this meant to you." He leans up to kiss you between the eyes. He continues but you blank out, watch his lips move. He is speckled in freckles, and you fixate on how they expand and contract around his mouth with each word.

"We'll get through this," he says.

Now the "we."

Joel turns on the faucet in the tub beside you.

"You're sure you're okay?"

"I don't want to go to the hospital."

Taking your words as gospel, one of his arms slinks under your legs, the other around your waist. The towel slips from your lap to the floor. It's a baptism. Your buttocks taste the bath water first. Joel angles his body and yours as he kneels, brings you into the liquid. You settle into the heat. It burns but it's a good hurt, a disinfecting type.

Joel twists away from you, grimaces at the toilet seat. He shuts the lid and reaches to flush.

"No!" You're suddenly mobile, thrusting out a hand to stop him.

Joel frowns. He stares at the toilet then back at you.

"You left the seat up again," you say.

Joel blinks a few times before saying, "What was that?"

"I ran in here. I fell in the toilet. Among other things my ass hurts."

"M, are you sure . . . about the hospital."

"Yes, I am sure. I am very, very *certain* I don't want to go to a hospital and answer questions that I'm sure you want to ask me right now. I don't want to talk about when my last period was or how many times this has happened or anything regarding my body. *Okay?*"

"Alright."

Joel sits you up like an invalid, and you allow his body to prop up yours. One hand soaps your back, the other pushes away the strands of hair webbed around your breasts. The ends of the scarf tied around your head dampen on your shoulders.

"Talk," you urge. His hands freeze on you. You regard him. He doesn't meet your eyes. He's about to speak. But you interrupt, say, "Talk about anything else but right now."

He answers after a bit. "About fifteen minutes before I was set to leave, I was paged. One of the junior residents flubbed with the tracheotomy kit." He shakes his head at the thought. You're five years removed from your first year, but Joel keeps you updated, his rants, his successes, his failures that he tries to hide when he comes home, his form alternating the heaviness of the mattress so much you can feel when a life has been lost on his shift.

"There was a good amount of blood," he stops. There's a buzzing that radiates off him like sound waves when he's had a good day. When patients straddle the line and he, or anyone, is able to make it a firm win. "I got a tube in just in time."

You remove the hand he has on your stomach and squeeze it under the water.

He continues, rushing through the rest, downplaying his shift. Joel's hand gets firmer washing your back. You take it, feel the scratch of a non-existent itch.

The real kicker is that at the time he was saving a life, you lost the hope for one. That drawbridge will be raised and shut, locking you on the outside, again. You press your hand against the wall, bite your lip, and hold in the groan not from cramps but from failure.

Joel pulls you in, darkening his scrubs, wetting the floor tiles. His eyes roam over your body in a way you haven't felt since you made the announcement to his family. He huffs or sighs or a mixture of the two. He gestures at your torso. "I hate seeing you in this much pain."

"This? This is nothing compared to what I hear childbirth is like."

Your husband asks if that was supposed to be a joke. The truth is, you don't even know.

*　*　*

The bedsheets were satin, as were the nightie you wore and the boxers Joel donned. The attempt at lovemaking turned into an exercise on how to stay *on* the bed. When you jumped atop satin on satin, centrifugal force slid you off in record time. At one point you were about to be in Joel's arms and the next your knees crashed against the wicker hamper stationed on the other side of the mattress. The marks of your descent were ashy scratches on your calves.

Joel fared better. He reached out to you as though ready to help you onto a fast-moving train while you ran alongside it. His whole face creased when he asked if you were alright. You laughed from the floor. Went into a fit that brought on tears and hiccups while you rubbed your leg. It was upon seeing you in hysterics that a grin broke on his face. Joel's arms were not enough against gravity or the fabric's smoothness and magnetism. You tried again, but writhing on your back midkiss, you, and Joel, slipped centimeter by centimeter until your feet touched the ground while Joel attempted to maintain a grip on the mattress.

Joel's exposed skin began to match the maroon of the spread. He cursed the wedding gift with each tug of a corner. "Screw." *Pull.* "These." *Yank.* "Sheets." *Rip.* Once bare, only the manufacturer's label apparent in a corner of the bed, did your husband lift you up then lay you on the mattress, moving on to work his tongue from your lips to your crevice.

Later, discarded of satin, he asked, "Who gave us that?"

"Mike."

"Of course," he said.

"We still have to write 'thank yous,'" you reminded him. The wedding had been a couple months ago. Towers of boxes filled with items of no real purpose were in the guest room adjacent to yours. One of the presents had been a melon baller.

"When," you'd asked your husband, "would I *ever* need this?"

"Maybe not 'need,' but it's handy to have isn't it?" was his response even though he also looked confused and more so concerned by the real estate being taken up in the space he had been lobbying for as his future office.

"Dear Mike, Thanks so much for the satin sheets and sleepwear. Joel and I enjoy slip-and-slide as a form of foreplay. Love, Joel and Mikayla Smith."

Joel brought you close, he on his side, you again on your back. "I like the sound of it."

"You want me to write that?"

"I like the sound of Joel and Mikayla Smith is what I meant."

"Oh," you turned your face to kiss his, getting more hair than head, "I do, too."

"It's disturbing he got us this." He gestured at the rejected boxers somewhere on the floor.

"What's disturbing is the color. It reminds me of blood."

You touched your stomach, sunken in from lying flat, but you puffed out your cheeks, another curve to add to the rest of you. "You know, I might be pregnant this time. Your little men could have already made a clear path to my thingamajig, and *boom,* baby."

"It's possible," he murmured, eyes shut. His hand atop your left breast was an opaque marker, a blanched patch against russet skin, looking as though he left it there while you were out in the sun.

"A girl, or a boy, would fit between us on this bed. Can you picture it? Wedged between us? Kicking and nuzzling." You thought on it. Attributed features to a not-yet-existent child. Curls, oak-toned skin, a mole, oval face, slim fingers. All of it from somewhere down the family line. A person come to being whom you would hold before revealing her (or him) to Joel, his family, your family, and saying, "See? See what a beautiful thing we made?"

Joel said he wasn't sure when he pushed his face through the curtain of your hair to kiss your neck again.

"You can't picture a hypothetical that will soon be a definite?" you asked.

"Can we simply luxuriate in the moment?"

You startled up, and Joel's hand dropped from your breast. Leaning on elbows, you said, possibly in an accusing manner, "What's that mean?"

He admitted, "I want to focus on the two of us right now."

"Don't kill the mood—"

"Maybe you're killing *mine,* M. Maybe—" Opening both eyes, Joel smiled, genuine and kind. "Neither of us are killing anything. Right?"

You squinted at him. Ready to whack him on the chest and hear the *smack* of your palm on his skin. "Don't treat me like a patient."

"I'm not."

"You *are.*"

He sat up then, trying to meet you ire for ire. "One night. One full night off in a *month* and I want to sit here with my *wife* and enjoy an evening alone. Of quiet. How it used to be between us before the wedding and the moving and all that other crap. I don't want to think about anything else but you and me. That's not wrong, M. And nothing you say will make me think I'm being unfair here."

Your lips faltered. To speak, to smile, to pout, to spew accusations?

"All I want, at this moment, is to know *we* want the same thing," you said.

Joel urged you down, resumed the placement of hands and face against your body. The spots where you touched were balmy while the rest of you cooled.

* * *

Joel is on his haunches beside the bathtub, his chest up not exuding authority so much but the appearance of strength. His arms rest against the tub's rim. When he breathes, his body lowers as though he's deflating. First you, now him.

"All this, it's not worth seeing you in pain."

You face the tile; you're growing to dislike the color the more you stare at it. "Childbirth, pregnancy, all of it, is pain. It's pain that leads to something good."

"This is happening so quickly this year. Maybe it's a sign—"

Arms open wide you show Joel his damaged prize. Water drips from your limbs and fingers, droplets glisten in the hair growing under your arms too damn quick. You shaved just the day before. "If anything, it's a sign something is wrong with me. God*damn* it." Your arms drop in the water splashing Joel and further dampening the rug underneath him. "I've worked for what everyone else wanted *for* me. Yet this, for some reason *this* is not happening."

Joel changes tactics, starts off in that tone again with, "I understand."

"You don't understand." Your fingers trail down his neck, the water dripping where your fingers glide. "You're still high off the fact that you averted a death tonight, so you cannot understand what I am feeling right now."

"You know what I understand?" Joel's voice fractures and goes soft, "I understand that the lining to your uterine wall broke down. That the egg and sperm didn't fuse chromosomes properly and come together in the way they should have. I *get* that this has happened before. I *get* that you want a child but this was not it." He motions with his head to the toilet. "It wasn't formed yet. It wasn't *ours*. And I get that there's nothing wrong with you. But do *you* understand that? Do you comprehend that this happens, *often?* Because *that,* that I understand."

Joel rises. He's taller than you but the feeling of being a weakling unable to move, the inability to have your body match the heat of your words while lying in dirty water leaves you at a significant disadvantage.

The bath and you have switched places, it's tepid, you warm. The blood spatters have dissolved into the water changing the overall hue. And you have changed, no longer an expectant mother. You're relegated back to woman, wife, the black lady lucky enough to snag the white doctor husband.

The reflection in the water isn't as clear as a mirror, but it's there and you can make out the eyes, the face, the contemplation around the edges of Joel whenever he's grasping at what to say. Joel bends toward you and offers his arm. The chill gets to you now that you're out of the water, along with the air and feeling hollowed out. You dig deep, stand up. You cross your arms covering your breasts.

Joel goes into husband mode and finds the right words: "We'll have a child."

"How do you know?" Anxiety surfaces of what you're not. You are *not* a doctor. You are *not* a success. You are *not* pregnant. You are *not* a daughter so much as an essence of someone who *could've* been more. "How do you know?" you ask Joel because someone has to have an answer so you can keep trying. Your body shakes from the cold, or the crush of reality racks you enough that your husband holds you upright with one arm.

He pulls your face to his and kisses you. A simple action that is supposed to solve everything; in a way it does and doesn't. "We will have a child because you deserve to be happy."

A towel lands around your shoulders. You tie it around you and tuck the corners of the cloth between your thighs. You wrap your hair within itself and tighten your scarf so it'll hold.

You gesture at your lower half. "I need to . . ."

"Yeah," he says. Joel's hands leave your face. His scent wafts off. He says he'll clean up the bedroom. "Take your time."

One leg steps out of the tub followed by the other. Your hand hovers over the flusher. There's a bit of release and a trickle starts on your inner thigh. Eyes closed, you lift up the lid swearing a creak sounds. You open one eye, easing the cover up more. Wondering if it's like the horror movies, a floating mass in liquid, webbed fingers, not whole though it had the possibility. The trickle works its way in a swirl around your leg down your inner knee. Another eye opens, the lid widens but a hand stops you setting it back down. The trail travels and pools in the middle of your toes. Your husband takes a hand in his and urges it to the flusher glistening in the light, the cleanest part of the bathroom at this very moment. Together you flick the handle down and the sound washes it away. A *whoosh* and a *gurgle* note it's done.

Untranslation

Kari Smalkoski

It hits you hardest when you aren't looking, when your guard is down and you're living your life. For example, you're at a picnic in your neighborhood park, chatting with your friendly neighbors as you watch your children play on the playground. As you discuss the upcoming school year, one of the mothers says to you, "When are you going to have more kids? Your son is growing up so fast. He needs a brother or sister." She then asks if you'd like to try the homemade salsa she whipped up while her youngest daughter was napping this morning. You appear aloof as you stare at your nails. A week later you're sitting in a meeting, and someone surprises everyone by bringing her newborn daughter with her. People take turns holding her, and you are overwhelmed by her new-baby smell combined with the faint scent of breast milk. Someone says, "I can't wait until it's my turn to hold her." You, on the other hand, feel as if someone punched you so hard in the stomach that nothing comes out when you try and speak.

You recall this same feeling in your body when you looked at a monitor with your infertility doctor who had helped you conceive your son. Now he's helped you conceive a second baby after over a year of infertility treatments. He was searching for this baby's heartbeat, wondering why she wasn't moving like last month when you saw her on the screen. You looked at her and knew she was gone. You likely knew before you had medical evidence. Just a month earlier, when you felt her moving, you told her that many mothers pregnant with their second babies have told you that they can't imagine loving this baby as much as they love their first child, but that you already know how deeply you love her, that you, her father, and brother have so much love to give. A couple of weeks later, when her moving stopped as did your lethargy, you knew something was different, but your heart and mind weren't ready to communicate about it. Your kind doctor told you, "I'm sorry, your baby is gone. There's no heartbeat anymore. I'm so sorry, Kari dear." He stood quietly with his head down and his hand on your shoulder while your husband held the lower half of your body, burying his face into your legs. Minutes later, your favorite nurse walked into the room crying, hugged you and didn't let go. In that moment, it was there, that feeling as if someone sucker punched you without warning and all you could do was wail, in the fetal position, but the room was completely silent.

In 2012, two and a half years after my miscarriage, I spent the summer in a Hmong village in Northern Thailand, conducting fieldwork for my dissertation. During this time, I told myself I would not get close to the family I stayed with, Joua and her only child, Mai, who was five. It seemed easy enough since Joua's English was limited, and my Hmong and Thai weren't much better than her English. Each morning, Mai woke me by pressing her sweet face against my mosquito net, giggling. I pressed my face up against hers and smiled sleepily, but happy that she was the first person I saw every day. I loved watching Joua and Mai together, loved the rhythm of their lives in their two-room house made of bamboo where they welcomed me in as if we were kin. I liked Joua immediately when I met her. We were both in our late thirties at the time and shared the same sense of humor. She was lovely, warm, and kind, never hesitating to help other women in the village. I knew that if we could speak the same language fluently, we would never run out of things to talk about, just like me and my girlfriends back home in Minneapolis.

In the evenings, the three of us watched Thai soap operas. The door remained wide open as a warm breeze gave us temporary relief from the thick July heat as we laughed, snacking on red licorice and occasionally yelling at a couple of dogs in the village who had roamed into the main room, which served as a living room, kitchen, and eating area. Mai reclined in her lawn chair, Joua lay on a blanket that covered part of the uneven, concrete floor, and I sat next to Mai. Some evenings we went to the market on Joua's motorbike as Mai sat in front, Joua sat in the middle driving, and I sat in back with my arms stretched out holding Mai's waist. With no air conditioning or windows in Joua and Mai's house, I relished the cool breeze of mountain air on my skin as Joua navigated her bike through several dirt roads, quickly buzzing by houses belonging to other Hmong clans.

At the market, Mai often grabbed my hand, and I held hers, surprised at how natural it felt to walk hand in hand with her. Women selling food in the market often remarked how pretty Mai was and that someday she would win a Hmong beauty pageant. Small plastic bags filled with prepared spicy ground pork, papaya salad, and purple sticky rice sat on tables, but Mai always guided me past them and asked me to buy her a tricolored tapioca dessert in a plastic cup, at which Joua scolded her, telling her to stop asking me, and purchased three cups of dessert for us to eat before heading back to the house. We often left as the sun set, the three of us connected to each other by a string of longing and love, holding one another tightly on Joua's motorbike. I enjoyed these evenings together immensely and wished we could ride around the village all night like that.

Back then, and sometimes now, little girls are challenging for me to be around. I tire easily with them, unlike boys, whose energy I will happily soak up on any given day. I need no invitation to get on the floor and wrestle with my son and his boy cousins. I love running and hiking with my son and his friends, playing sports with them, and promoting books to them I think they will like. I've settled into a comfortable narrative that I'm just a mom who was meant to have a boy. We all wear armor in one form or another; mine is the neat and tidy identity I've constructed as a boy-mom.

Each morning after breakfast, Mai caught a bus to a private school outside of the village, and I left to do fieldwork. On days when I returned early, I'd see Joua on the same blanket in the middle of the floor, holding her legs to her chest, watching Thai soap operas without Mai and me. Her sadness was palpable. Once I found her crying, holding a picture. In the evenings, after Mai fell asleep, I listened as she talked in almost a whisper to her husband, using international calling cards and a cell phone that she had purchased at the 7-Eleven with money he wired her from South Korea. Much of this money was spent on Mai's schooling, which they believed would give her opportunities to leave the village for college. Like many men in the village with young children, Mai's husband had been away for over two years as a foreign laborer. She sang love songs to him and sounded half her age when she talked with him. When Mai was home, this side of her was absent, but I knew she was grieving for a man she feared she would never see again and whom she loved deeply.

One evening, I was given a Hmong name and adopted into Joua and Mai's clan. After the naming took place at her sister-in-law's house, Joua had me cut herbs in their garden for dinner. "You eat these herbs tonight, and when you go home to America you'll get pregnant with a girl. When you come back to visit us, she'll be with you," Joua told me as she piled the boiled herbs on my plate next to the chicken she had killed and cooked for the occasion. All of the women in the clan said I had to have a daughter because I'd already been blessed with a son. I didn't tell them I'd already lost my chance at having a daughter or the words of the nurse who called a couple of weeks after my miscarriage. "The fetus was a girl. If you have any questions, follow up with your doctor." *Click.*

I've got no punchy comeback lines when people remind me that I'm too old to give my son a sibling. Just recently a family member remarked that I should be grateful that I only have one child because my life is infinitely less complicated than those of the women in my family who have two or more. The truth is, I've never feared getting older, it's just easier and more digestible to tell everyone that I'm in the midst of a forty-something midlife crisis, instead of discussing the reason behind the crisis. There are nights when I hold my son as he sleeps and can't stop the waves of sadness followed by guilt that wash over me. Get over it, I say to myself, you have him. Move on. It has been several years now. After my miscarriage, I received immeasurable support from women who were already part of this club that nobody wants to be a member of. One of them told me to prepare myself for the hurtful things people would inevitably say to me, but she didn't warn me about the judgmental things I would say to myself.

A friend tells me that the experiences we have in other countries are untranslatable. I think this also applies to miscarriage. It is hard to describe what it's like to lose someone I never saw outside of my body, never held, never grew to know or love, but whom I felt intimately attached to and who was already connected to my husband and son. As a Korean adoptee, raised in a white family, I longed to have babies that were related to me. I could only imagine what it would be like to finally look at another person's face and see myself reflected back. When I miscarried, I experienced yet another loss of a person who was a part of me. It is challenging to articulate and impossible to find words in any language to describe what it's like to long for a family that was supposed to be, when I am grateful for and fiercely love the family I have. It is the incompleteness that I struggle with. It is missing someone I never knew, but whom I wanted desperately to be a part of my life.

The day I left the village to fly to Bangkok, Joua was busy making breakfast, so I brushed Mai's long hair and put it up in barrettes like she wore it to school. She sat in her Thai school uniform, at her pink plastic table near my makeshift bed, and decorated her Barbie ruler-lined notebook with princess stickers I'd brought her from the United States. We took selfies together with my camera. In each one we are laughing with our cheeks pressed together and her arms are wrapped around my neck. Early before breakfast, she'd been playing with other children in the village. I watched as a small posse of boys and girls followed her around the dirt paths between houses as she made plans and gave them tasks to carry out in their imaginary world. As I brushed her long hair, I thought about how my daughter would have had long black hair too and that no matter how much I would try and steer her away from all things pink, princess, and telling other kids what to do, that's the sort of daughter I imagine I would have had. As Joua and I embraced several times before I left, she said in tears, "I wish you never had to leave us. All of our meals taste so much better with you here."

On the small plane I flew in to Bangkok, I put my suitcase into the overhead bin and then realized I had been assigned a seat across the aisle from a little girl and her mother. I saw them at the gate at the airport and noticed the girl's father was sitting behind me. I turned around and said to him, "Hey, do you want to switch seats so you can sit across from your family?" He smiled and said in a thick French accent, "Thank you. That is very kind." We switched seats quickly, and his daughter and wife turned around and exclaimed happily in unison, "Thank you!" His wife was Asian, and their daughter, half Asian, a *hapa,* like my son, reached for her father's hand across the aisle and never let go until the plane was above the clouds. She and her mother, both beautiful with long black hair like my own, held hands the entire flight. Every now and then she turned around to look at me and study the dress I was wearing, my shoes, and my purse. When I smiled at her, she smiled back shyly and looked away.

Sometimes she and her father spoke together in French as her big brown eyes grew with excitement about whatever they talked about. When the one-hour flight landed in Bangkok, her father handed me my suitcase from the overhead bin, and we wished one another farewell. I thought of my own family of three as they walked together, hand in hand, to baggage claim. Once I was in a taxi, I saw them standing nearby at the curb, waiting for a ride. I looked at the girl, who appeared to be around my son's age, chatting with her parents. And as my taxi pulled away from the curb, I watched them watch me, until we were all out of sight.

Flunking Math

Arfah Daud

Except for my black leather backpack,
shoes, and the dark preserves that stained
my underwear, I was dressed in solid white
the day I flunked my algebra test.
I accepted my failure.
Palms placed against the wall,
I pushed hard against the pain.
My mother and the lies she told of how easy birth was.
God stretching the vagina like an elephant's.
That particular evening, the sky was dark gray,
and the sun bled the sky crimson.
My mother, miscarrying in the bathroom
of that old rented house, calling and calling for my father.
The child, a fish-like form on the wet floor,
its black opened eyes gazed blankly at me.
I walked over to Mr. John's office to go over the test.
He said math is easy. One plus one plus one is easy
I thought but I get confused with algebra.
In algebra substitute a number for x and y.

It's okay to fail Mr. John said and my eyes welled up.
I had miscalculated.

    I pushed my head back
and howled. This is what they looked like, the others
that I had decided to let go. Each time I'd grab
the doctor's hand in gratitude.
I could have fitted the length of each fish-like
form nicely in the palm of my hand.

Returning to Morro Bay

Arfah Daud

Hemlock Ave, January 21st

Walking silently down that same quiet street
I stopped where the small house
used to be, where my life began in a new country.

In this small city the fog on summer evenings lingered.
Giant pine trees, dramatic limbs black
against the small cottage, shadowed
the tall houses on the street.

Standing there alone, I hear waves
pounding the shore,
listen for echoes of my children's footsteps
as they drifted in one after the other from school,
and for what might have been . . .

A new house, bigger, double story,
rests on the tiny grave.

Avenue of Poplars in Autumn

Arfah Daud

After Van Gogh for my mother

In Autumn, Vincent's poplars' fiery leaves, lustrous;
burnt orange, ocher, orange like flames
gradually turn to brown piled up in heaps on the ground.
In the flickering light, lines of trees throw shadows
leading to the wooden house where young women,
married or single, would come and go frequently.
They go in frightened, they come out hollowed
and filled with more fear.

In the faces of these women, you'd see their desperation.
The promises they made, which we all know no one keeps.
So, they go back again and again to the house in the woods.
To the old wooden table, the kitchen scattered with empty bottles
and old flasks, the soft light like weak tea, and to the young
cassava shoots whittled down to a tool, sharp as a needle.

Night arrives trailing the crimson sky. The cloaked woman
walks home alone leaving greyish black shadows behind.

Slowly she walks clutching the void in her belly. Regret
is my mother telling me the number of children she could have had.
Of unmarked stones scattered around the house.
Of wind-whipped leaves making sounds of babies crying
in the yard of that house in the woods.

Sianneh

The Trip Was Good

Shannon Gibney

Monica's brow is furrowed in concentration, but also worry, I see now. She has me hooked up to a fetal monitor to measure the baby's heartbeat. I am seated upright on a faux leather examination table. Two flat sensors stretch across my belly and attach back to a machine with leads and buttons and lights. She tried the Doppler fetal monitor we normally use when we first came into the birthing room, but then switched over to this more complicated one.

"What's wrong?" I ask tentatively.

Ballah sits on the small couch across from me, completely absorbed in his phone.

Monica frowns. "I can't quite find the baby's heartbeat."

Something catches in my throat. "What?"

Monica's eyes meet mine furtively, but I can't begin to understand what I'm seeing. She has been one of my three primary midwives these past nine months and is a competent, warm woman, but I still don't know her that well. She puts her small, white hand on mine. "Don't get worried yet. She's probably just hiding. Sometimes they need some encouragement. Let me get you some fruit juice, which should get everything moving, okay?"

I nod, because I don't know what else to do.

Monica rushes out of the room, and suddenly everything is quiet. It is dusk, and the light through the leaves on the trees outside makes them look almost like birds' wings through the windows. Someone in the upscale St. Paul neighborhood honks a horn down the street. I burst into tears.

"Babe?" Ballah asks.

"Didn't you hear her?" I am trying to wipe the tears away as fast as they are falling. "They can't find the baby's heartbeat."

He looks at me in confusion. I am sure he doesn't know what this means, what it could mean.

"But . . ." He turns to look out the door, down the hallway. "Where did she go?"

I reach down and pull a Kleenex from the box on the small dresser beside me. "She went to get some fruit juice for me to drink. Hopefully, the sugar will get the baby moving more, so that it's easier to pick up her heartbeat."

He nods. "Okay."

But I know he still doesn't grasp the full implications. He isn't worried. Not like me.

He is seated on a bright-yellow divan about two feet away from me. I grab his hand, impulsively. "It's going to be okay, right babe?" I want him to reach out to me, to hug me and rub my back.

"Yes," he says stiffly. He stands beside me, completely contained in his own body. The only part of him touching me is his right hand. "Yes, it will be okay."

"Okay," I say, squeezing his hand. Maybe this way, I can make it be true.

Monica runs back up the stairs and hands me a small bottle of apple juice. I feel nauseous and don't want to drink it at all, but force it down. Afterwards, she turns the machine back on, and the sensors still hum softly, recording nothing.

"We're going in," she says to me then. "We're going to the hospital. We don't have an ultrasound machine here, and we need to know what's happening. Amy's bringing the car around."

Amy is the head midwife at the birthing center, the woman who brought Boisey, my son, into the world at my house three and a half years ago. If Monica has called her in now, at the very beginning of labor, something must really be wrong. Hot tears sting the corners of my eyes, and I wince as a contraction comes over me.

Monica and Ballah help me down the stairs, and Amy screeches the car to a stop on the curb. "Get her in quickly," she tells them. "There's no time to waste."

She drives like a maniac all the way to Regions Hospital in downtown St. Paul, swerving through turns, almost running lights. The world on the other side of the car windows goes by in a blur, and I myself do not feel real. I feel gelatinous, a bit like putty, neither solid nor liquid. Like I no longer have edges to contain me.

"Has anything like this ever happened to you before?" I ask Amy as we wait for the last light to change.

I see her grimace through her profile. "Just once before," she says. She has delivered more than 350 healthy babies, so that is something.

"How did it turn out?" I ask carefully. I know she will not lie to me.

She grimaces again. "Honestly, not well, Shannon."

I nod. I don't want to know any more.

When we reach the hospital, they pull up a wheelchair and make me sit in it.

"But I can walk," I say, but they shake their heads.

They wheel me down several winding hallways, with bright fluorescent lights, and photos of lakes with cranes and geese. I try to steady my breathing, which I can feel is irregular. Finally, we come to the OB-GYN ward, and they hurry me into one of the patient rooms. Ballah is instructed to sit in the waiting room. An ultrasound machine, which I have been hooked up to many times before for routine checkups, sits beside the bed in my room.

"We're just going to see what's going on," says a doctor, looking me carefully in the eyes. She appears be in her late thirties, like me, and her thin blonde hair is pulled to the nape of her neck in a black plastic clasp.

I nod.

I don't want to be here.

I lie down on the bed.

The doctor sits on the chair beside me. She squirts some transmission fluid on my raised stomach, and an image of a baby lying on her back, feet up, comes onto the screen. The baby is not moving. The baby has no heartbeat.

Two more doctors come into the room and stand next to Amy, who is seated in the corner.

"Okay," says the doctor with the ultrasound probe. "So, yes. The baby has no heartbeat." She puts the ultrasound probe down and stands up.

I look from her back to the screen, and the baby still isn't moving. "Okay," I say. I want to ask her how to get the heartbeat started again, but some part of my brain is telling me not to say that.

"I'm sorry," she says. "I'm so sorry."

I look to Amy, then each of the three doctors beside her. Discomfort drains their faces, though I can see they are trying hard to mask it. I wonder how it feels to have to tell a woman something like that and then still be expected to remain professional. It must not be easy. I ask if I can go to the bathroom.

Once inside the bathroom, I grip the sink until my knuckles are white, and stare into the spotless mirror. The woman looking back at me has dark-brown eyes that hold nothing. What was once a sharp chin is now round and plump. Her hair frizzes all over from the humidity. I turn on the faucet as high as it will go, and flush the toilet. Then I scream. The woman in the mirror screams and lets go of the sink as she does it. She wonders if she is just a copy of herself today, and if her real self is back at home, washing dishes. She does not want to go back into the patient room, because she knows they will tell her what she has to do next, and she does not want to know what she has to do next. She does not want to leave the bathroom, because she will have to say to her husband, *Our baby is dead*. She does not want to call her mother, because her mother will cry, and nothing will make her stop. She does not like to see or hear her mother cry. She will have to rewrite the story of the pregnancy, and the baby coming, the happy house, her young son so eager to be a brother. Now the story will center on a chapter in which the eagerly awaited baby dies in utero, never to be cuddled and warmed in her arms, never to scream and demand a diaper change, never to suckle her breast. The woman does not want that story. She is not ready for it, for what it will mean—not just now, today, tonight, but forever, for the rest of her life. The weight of that story could crush all other stories of her life and the lives of those she loves. She does not want that. She is too tired, and she wants to sleep. She wants to awaken.

I place my hand on my belly and tell my baby I love her. Then I open the door. I shuffle slowly back to the room, telling myself this is real with every step.

"What do I have to do?" I ask them, back in the room. I have just had another contraction, and the force of it stuns me into a chair beside the door. "Why did it happen?"

The head doctor, I will learn later that her name is Dr. Richardson, winces. I feel sorry for them, having to deal with this, deal with me. I am quite sure they didn't become doctors or midwives in order to comfort and care for pregnant women with dead babies inside them. What could they possibly say or do to comfort or care for anyone in this situation?

"You're already in labor, right?" Dr. Richardson asks me.

I nod.

"She's in the very early stages," says Amy.

Dr. Richardson nods. "Then my recommendation would be to just let it develop and give birth to the baby vaginally."

The rest of the doctors murmur their agreement.

I blink once, then again. I stare at Dr. Richardson, and then Amy in the eyes. "You mean I still have to go through labor? With a dead baby?" The ice on my words cuts everyone in the tiny room.

"Yes," Amy says quietly.

"Can't you cut it out of me or something?" I ask. "What is the point?"

"This is really hard. Really hard. But the safest way to get the baby out is still through vaginal birth," says Dr. Richardson.

"Not safest for her," I say quietly. "My uterus was obviously not safe."

"We still don't know what happened. And unfortunately, the truth is that we may never know," says Dr. Richardson. Later, I will learn that close to half of all stillbirths in the United States are never accounted for. No one knows why the baby died. "But this doesn't mean that your uterus isn't safe. Or at least as safe as anyone else's." She looks away from me for a moment and then settles her dark-brown eyes back on mine. "But yes, I meant safest for you." She fiddles with her hair clasp, and I feel a pang of guilt for making her answer things that cannot be answered, to direct anger that has no place to go. Still, I cannot help myself.

"How long will it take?" I ask. "For her to come out?"

"It's hard to know," says Amy. "Sometimes it goes faster in situations like this, sometimes it's the same amount of time."

"Okay," I say. I want to awaken. "Can I tell my husband what's going on?"

The doctors and Amy nod. They tell me they're going to move me upstairs to a birthing room.

When I walk into the waiting room, Ballah is seated by the door, staring into space. Kathleen, my dear friend and doula, sits beside him.

"It's dead," I say when I am about twenty feet away from them. I am not shouting, but I am definitely talking louder than I need to. I want everyone in the waiting room and at the nurses' station to hear. "The baby inside me is dead."

Ballah doesn't say anything.

"What? I don't understand," Kathleen says. She stands up and walks to hug me, and I allow it, though I am stiff.

The hospital staff rush behind me with the wheelchair and start to wheel me down the hall. I get the feeling that they want me out of there as fast as possible. It would be bad if innocent and unsuspecting pregnant women knew exactly what could happen to their beloved babies, no matter how unlikely.

Once I am in the birthing room, everyone is called: my parents, my friends, Ballah's family. Amy and Monica stay with me while I pace between contractions that seem to blissfully wipe out my consciousness every few minutes, in tsunami after tsunami of pain. A nurse comes in to monitor my vitals from time to time, quietly and expertly tending to me, her patient.

"Will I be able to have another baby after this?" I ask Monica, between clenched teeth.

She nods, sadly. Her pale face is streaked with red, and I realize that she must have been crying one of those times that she stepped out of the room. "Yes," she says. "You can definitely have another baby."

I nod back at her. But the knowledge does not even give me the semblance of peace. "Oh!" I shudder, as another contraction reverberates through me. I run into the bathroom, a blinding need to defecate pulling me.

I stand over the toilet, contemplating something—anything—coming out to relieve the pressure. The two female doctors who were in the ultrasound room suddenly rush in, asking me what's wrong. "I think I have to take a shit!" I sob. Something like fire is bearing down on my bottom and my vagina simultaneously. I think that if I do not expel it now, I will explode.

"Well, it's probably your baby!" exclaims one doctor.

The other one maneuvers around me so that my right foot is perched on the toilet flusher. Then the first doctor crouches below my vagina, as I start to push.

Later, Ballah will tell me that he wept, outside in the hallway, hearing me scream as I pushed her out of me. "All that pain," he will say, stroking my hair at home in our bed. "All of it for nothing."

But he is wrong, because when she comes out, she is perfect. Long and thin and mopped with curly brown hair just like her brother, I can see that there is nothing wrong with her, that there could never be anything wrong with my perfect, silent daughter. We named her "Sianneh," which means "The Trip Was Good," in Loma, the language of Ballah's ethnic group back home in Liberia. "Sianneh, the trip was good," Kathleen will say to me later, stroking my arm delicately as a small group of close friends surround me. "The trip is always good." A tear will escape from the side of my eye before I can stop it, and I will wipe it away quickly with the back of my hand. But right now, the doctors delicately lead me to the hospital bed, holding her carefully, as if she is breathing. When I lie down, pillows propped against the back of me so I can sit up, they hand her to me. I cradle her in my arms and gaze at her, so exhausted. So elated. So destroyed.

Binding Signs

Dania Rajendra

I discovered, much to my shock and chagrin, that I wanted a baby of
my own in the back of an auto-rickshaw. It was June 2008. It was sunny,
warm, comfortable as it usually is in Mysore, India. I sat in the rickshaw
with my cousin and her two-year-old, which by Indian familial logic
makes her my niece. I'm Indian on my father's side—he immigrated in
1970. I'm Jewish on my mother's—she's from the Bronx. I visit my family
in India often, and as my cousin and her daughter and I bumped along in
the sunshine, the reddish dust (deforestation is but one legacy of British
colonialism) puffed around us, mixing with the diesel exhaust. My niece
napped against me, her squishy body slowly turning solid as she passed
from dozing to sleeping. I held her tightly enough to keep her inside the
moving vehicle, loosely enough so she could sleep undisturbed. I can no
longer remember where we were going, or why. I just remember a new
need crawled out of my heart and took up residence in my solar plexus. I
had to remind myself to breathe.

That June, I was six months into my first marriage; my husband and I
had a shared ambivalence about whether we wanted children. We were
leftist activists. He was in law school, I was in creative writing school and
working full-time. We had a lot we wanted to do with ourselves—travel,

make change, have fun. Maybe, we thought, our lives would be full enough without kids.

I returned from India—an extended visit with my *ajji* (grandmother in Kannada), my aunts and uncles, my cousins—and resumed my life in New York. Six months later, my husband and I agreed, we'd start trying. He'd be almost done with law school. I'd be turning thirty.

We tried. He graduated. I got a new job. We tried. He got a postgraduate fellowship, then a new one, in Baltimore. We tried. We moved. We tried some more. It was six months, it was twelve, it was eighteen. People advised us to relax, which just pissed us off. We decided to go on vacation, yes, to relax and also to get away from people telling us to relax. Our options for a last-minute December trip—close to the East Coast, beachy—included Panama, El Salvador, Mexico, Puerto Rico, Costa Rica. The latter won out.

Whenever we went on vacation in Latin America, the same thing always happened. Because I look Latina (brown, with dark hair) and my husband is tall, blue-eyed, fair-haired, people would always address me in Spanish. But he's the one who speaks the language. In Costa Rica, our plans were to surf, eat tropical fruits, and drink cocktails. But we discovered I was pregnant. I needed my husband to teach me how to say "pregnant" in Spanish, to read the labels on painkillers, the words to refuse uncooked vegetables, raw fruit, alcohol, coffee. I used my phone to check BabyCenter, which told me my embryo was the size of a lentil. We began to make plans, talk names, dream. And, then, a couple of days later, I got really, really sick. Maybe it was the food? Maybe it was the flu? I stayed in bed for a couple of days, shooing my husband out to surf, drink cocktails, and eat fresh fruit without me. When I started to bleed, we drove to the hospital in Puntarenas. Even though it was my husband who spoke Spanish, it was me who made sense of the words from the doctor: *Trompa de Fallopia. Ectópico. Emergencia.*

The doctor made sure to explain to us that it wasn't an abortion, because the pregnancy wasn't viable. *Viable* is the same in English and Spanish. What he said was, "It's not a sin." He said it over and over. Neither of us told him I was Jewish, feminist, not Catholic. Neither of us told him we're for abortion on demand, without apology. Neither of us told him much of anything.

Because we were Americans with good insurance and a healthy credit card limit, we took the calculated risk the doctor recommended: drive to the capital for laparoscopic surgery at the private hospital. "Go now," he told us, "and don't stop for any reason." He said that, repeatedly, in Spanish and then in English. Don't stop. For any reason. If my tube burst, I could hemorrhage to death in the car. "But you should be okay." It was the middle of the night.

The hospital in Puntarenas was the only place we went in Costa Rica that wouldn't take U.S. dollars. My husband had to go find Costa Rican currency, while I paced in the payment office, humming the same tune over and over again. I was surprised to realize it was "Avinu Malkeinu." It was soothing, so I hummed it, quietly, bent over in pain, until my husband came back with the money.

He got behind the wheel, I climbed into the passenger seat. He steered us onto the highway to San José, pushed his foot all the way down on the accelerator, and he asked me the same questions over and over, to keep me awake, so he would know I wasn't passed out from internal bleeding. It's usually a two-hour drive. I think he made it in forty-five minutes.

The next day a surgeon removed my lentil-sized embryo and the fallopian tube it was stuck in. Left to grow, the embryo that I wanted so badly to be my first child would have killed me. As a person of Indian descent, I'm familiar with lentils of many kinds and all sizes: fresh, dried, whole, split. Even now, ten years later, when I wash lentils, I pinch the thin discs between my fingers and marvel that the tiny potential of a person can be packed into such a small package.

Soon after our not-very-relaxing vacation, we moved to Mississippi, where citizens had just voted down personhood legislation, which might have outlawed my life-saving surgery and certainly would have banned the IVF we tried. I thought, often, of the Costa Rican doctor: "It's not a sin." I was grateful, deeply, that we had vacationed in Costa Rica instead of El Salvador, which has banned the surgery that saved my life, and instead women in my situation must wait for the tube to rupture before doctors can attempt the measures that might save their lives. Even Hinduism, which is stricter than Judaism on this subject, recognizes the priority of the life of the mother over the life of the embryo.

The different ideas my husband and I had of what the embryo had been—a "person," or, as Jewish law suggests, not—and how to grieve the loss, exacerbated our existing tensions. I admired much about Mississippi and the people I met there, but it was hard to live in such a thoroughly Christian place, with so little space for me as a not-black, not-white person. My white, Southern husband couldn't feel the same squeeze I did. Infertile, far from friends and family in a place unwelcoming, I imagined that my tube, fished out by the doctor, had magically regenerated as a tiny glass pipette containing outer space: cold, dark, pricked by teeny, tiny stars. No matter how hot and humid Mississippi got, I never felt warm.

My IVF attempt spanned the fall, Thanksgiving, and Christmas. Everywhere in Jackson was decorated to welcome the little baby son of God. I felt trapped, sometimes I felt my whole self had been subsumed into that glass tube of space. I went, once, to a support group. Unlike the other women in it, there was no easy blanket of religious tradition for me. I'm from a family where religious observance consisted of latkes at Hanukkah and politics over the seder table—in part because that's what we did, and in part because our mixed-race, atheist family with radical politics wasn't welcome in 1980s-era New York suburban synagogues. I only knew "Avinu Malkeinu" because I had started to go to shul on the High Holy Days with friends in college. I had always yearned for more, though, and when we agreed to try for a child, I figured I'd find my way when I became a Jewish mother of a Jewish child. (My husband did not want to convert but agreed we'd raise our child Jewish.) I found little comfort in Internet-based pregnancy loss forums, awash with alienating talk of angels that failed to speak to my own pro-choice, Jewish, and Hindu understandings. So I tried the support group—once. I never went back, though, because of politics—the politics of personhood. After an awkward conversation around a table at a room in the library, I found myself exiting the parking lot, my car behind one of the other ladies. My headlights illuminated her pro-Personhood bumper sticker. I felt sick, and not only from the hormones.

My Christian in-laws called often with positive thinking, encouraging voice mails. It wasn't their fault, but it pissed me off. I found myself holding the rational positions about the unlikelihood of its success (IVF cycles fail 60 to 80 percent of the time) as a bulwark. The faith that comforted my in-laws, my neighbors, the people on the Internet, it grated on me. I began to dig into Jewish texts to understand what the teachings offer about what embryos are and how to make sense of "bad luck" in general. I began to bake challah on Fridays. It felt like the only way to find a space to live like a person, as the Yiddish expression has it. Just after Christmas, my IVF failed.

It's not unusual for infertility to strain a marriage. It's common that infertility makes people feel lonely. My first husband is a good, deeply feeling man, but we were mired in our own, very different experiences— our own childhoods, our own cultural and personal ideas of what it meant not to be able to conceive and what it meant to lose the embryos. For him, I think, they are children. I think he believes that, and I think his family does, too. When he called my father-in-law from Costa Rica after the surgery to share the news that I had been pregnant and was no longer, my father-in-law said, "For a little while, I was a grandfather." My parents did not say such things. They focused less on the embryo, more on me. My mother said, "It's sad, but it's not tragic. Your dying would have been tragic." In all that, there's so little room for ambivalence.

But ambivalence is a part of grief and of infertility. For me, infertility provoked another internal conflict: embryos are not people, and yet, I have missed the people those embryos never became every day since I lost them. I expect to for the rest of my life, even as I am certain there is no such thing as a "good" abortion—the kind society says I had—or a "bad" one. All I know is that I walk around in a warm and living body that carries a brittle length of something hollow, full of dark, cold, missing person-potential.

I worked out my ambivalence in many ways: I volunteered at the last remaining abortion clinic in Mississippi, conveniently around the corner from our house. I stopped going to baby showers. I retreated into Jewish tradition, where the comfort with conflict and ambivalence felt like the only place to grapple with these questions, even as organized Jewish life can be forbidding and family oriented. It was hard to find a way to observance, especially in Mississippi (though there are Jews there, of course), so my ways were small, and personal, and contained by our house, in which lived just one Jew and one person whose atheist sensibilities didn't really allow for observance without belief. So I felt I had to tiptoe toward observance and kept my Jewish curiosity to myself, reading more and talking less. I baked bread, I lit candles, but I said no blessings, and I sang no tunes. I did begin to seethe about how my white husband, like all my white boyfriends before him, was more into my Indianness than my Jewishness. Indian was exotic, strange, and erotic. Think the Kama Sutra, whispery silk saris, food studded with nuts and lentils and chili and cumin. In the lefty cultures we inhabit, being a person of color (and, sometimes, being married to one) confers a certain, unassailable authority on race and, in the case of Indians, colonialism. Jewishness does not, associated as it is with American elites, complicated international problems, stinky fish products—none of which were particularly sexy or interesting. We lived in the same house but began to inhabit separate worlds. Finally, we returned home to Brooklyn. Our marriage fell apart. Freed, adrift, I began to attend shul on Saturday mornings.

Shabbat services—the practice of joy—were just what I needed to find a small measure of peace in the maelstrom of infertility, divorce, and my father's terminal lung cancer. I was desperately grateful that all of me—my lefty politics, my lack of Jewish knowledge, my atheism, my mixed-race, mixed-heritage identities—were welcome at shul.

When my father died, I clung again to Judaism's mourning rituals. Shabbat became a container for the immensity of my feelings, a time to sit inside my grief and to embrace new joy as it came. After the first month of mourning ended, I went to India, the first extended visit since I had discovered, years before, that I wished to be a mother. There, I continued keeping Shabbat in my family's house. Generally, alcohol is shunned in observant Brahmin households, but every week, my uncle took me to buy wine. Every week, my *ajji,* my aunt, and my uncle listened as I blessed the tiny oil lamps I borrowed from the pooja room, I blessed the wine, I blessed the slice of white bread from the local bakery and dipped it in salt, and handed it around. They chewed as I recited Kaddish. (My uncle shared in the wine; my *ajji* and my aunt did not.) My grandmother told me how glad she was I had something to do, that I was doing some ritual of remembrance, of grief, of recognition, even as it was not hers. It was a special thing to share—a current of feeling, expressed so differently.

I returned again to New York. To mark my exit from those years of sorrow, I ran the New York City marathon, cheered on by a new love. I also hired a Hebrew tutor. At her suggestion, I ran loop after loop in Prospect Park to the v'ahavta, learning the sounds, the rhythm, and, in some way, inscribing the might of the prayer into muscle memory. On marathon day, I jogged through Hasidic Williamsburg slowly, sounding out the signs, propelled by my new ability to read Hebrew letters—aided, in no small part, by my previously hard-won ability to read Kannada letters. As I jogged along slowly, I considered the homes in which I was simultaneously inscribing the words. The home of my body, with which I was slowly making peace in it-is-never-making-a-baby-love-it-anyway form. The home I was constructing of Jewish ritual. It was the Jewish imperative of joy that helped me find air when I felt I might drown in a vast vacuum of sadness. It was Jewish ritual that gave me the courage to grab strong hold of my new love, my *bashert,* who somewhat unbelievably is also Indian and Jewish, also leftist, also finds pickled fish and political arguments sexy and romantic.

Braided, our similarities (we both love country music), our differences (he's a planner; I'm not), our affection—those strands make us a family, complete in the two of us. Some days, I feel unbelievably lucky. Some days, my sorrow that we will not make yet another curly-haired, Indian-Jewish-lefty little human is boundless. It pushes out of its imaginary glass vial, exceeds its brittle boundaries, seeps cold into my bones. But most days, that is not my main problem. Most days, my problems are the usual marathon of everyday American adult life: Overly long commutes. Irritating coworkers. Political setbacks and advances. Insufficient funds for the things I prefer to do. That everydayness is a blessing, a binding sign of the fullness of this life—my life—and its importance unto itself. In the throes of infertility, it felt like my whole life orbited my inability to conceive, to bring forth a new person, the grief and the longing. It is hard work to keep that dark, cold feeling to its proper size and scope— acknowledged and contained. Every week, as my new husband and I welcome Shabbat with blessings we recite aloud, the regular rhythm of Jewish ritual is a reminder: my life matters more than my lost embryos'. Maybe in another ten years I won't need the reminder. In the meantime, I am glad for the sign, and I inscribe it upon my doorpost.

Massimo's Legacy

Diana Le-Cabrera

When we found out we were pregnant for the first time, we were absolutely over the moon. After being together for eight years, we tied the knot. Luis and I had been building our lives together for so long that we finally felt that it was the right time to start trying. We didn't register for wedding gifts but rather asked guests to contribute to a honeymoon fund because we didn't need anything—we wanted more memories. Our two-week vacation to Spain, Bulgaria, Greece, and Italy was unforgettable. About a month after coming home, still on a high, we found out we were pregnant. Well actually, I, of course, found out first. I honestly didn't think it could happen so fast and was a little worried how Luis might react. Instead, I saw pure joy in his face. We felt so blessed to expand our family the same year we married—it was like a fairy tale, too good to be true.

We knew about friends who had had miscarriages, so like many couples, we waited until after the first trimester to tell loved ones. It worked out so well that our immediate families were traveling into town for Thanksgiving, for it was right after our nuchal translucency scan. We had passed the first trimester, had ultrasounds to share, and learned that we were at the lowest risk for certain genetic issues. We couldn't wait to share what we were thankful for this year!

We planned it so that when Luis said grace, he would announce that we had a blessing brewing in my belly. Everyone was raising their wineglasses, in prayer and thanks, and I was anxiously awaiting—but he didn't tell them. There I was with my wineglass full of apple cider thinking, "Well, now what?" while trying not to look suspicious. I did the best I could to play host, and finally, before dessert was served, he started to share, first in Spanish. My mother-in-law actually interrupted his announcement, shouting, "Bebé!" My parents looked around confused. I'm not quite sure how they didn't make the connection that *bebé* sounds like *baby,* but it didn't take long for them to realize once Luis shared the announcement in English. My mother-in-law already suspected when she saw me pour cider instead of wine. Our families cheered and clinked their wineglasses so much that we were almost invisible during their celebration. We tried to ask them if they wanted to see the ultrasounds, but they were busy congratulating themselves on becoming uncles and aunts and grandparents! It was the best Thanksgiving yet.

I was a jolly, calm mother who loved the pregnancy process. I was lucky in that I was just mildly nauseous, and the only physical discomforts I had were carpal tunnel and swelling. I didn't even consider my first-trimester exhaustion as troublesome, because I love to sleep. Instead, when someone asked me about the discomforts of my pregnancy, I replied that the biggest one was actually the election of Donald Trump.

For the first time when voting, I didn't think about my future family in an abstract manner. I felt even more strongly about choosing the candidate who would help build a better future for my children. I was worried for my son, who would be biracial—half Dominican and half Vietnamese—given the political dividedness of our nation. Luis was an immigrant who came from the Dominican Republic, and I was first-generation Vietnamese American. We both grew up in humble homes with loving parents who did the best they could to show us a better life than they had had back in their third-world countries. We had experienced our share of profiling and racism, and my first child was going to be born into a world where he would already be judged and deemed less to some folks solely by his looks and his name.

As the initial poll results came in, I recall being optimistic. Even as the last state poll results were displayed on the TV, I stared at them in denial, truly thinking that I would wake up on November 5, 2017, and Hillary Clinton would be president. Luis, more realistic, didn't say a word and quietly went to sleep. He shared the next day that he wasn't surprised, just immensely disappointed. He looked at me and promised me that no matter who was president, we were going to have to fight for our family and prepare ourselves as best as we could. I sobbed on the phone with my best friend, who assured me that she would help show my son that this world can be kind and open-minded. Just like our parents did with us, I dreamed of a future where he wouldn't have to struggle as much as Luis and I did.

This desire fueled my encouragement of Luis to pursue his developer dreams. He wanted to attend a part-time boot camp for the second half of my pregnancy but was hesitant to leave me mostly alone for twenty weeks. It would mean that he would work his normal nine-to-five and then go to the boot camp afterwards. He would return home around nine thirty Monday through Thursday and have projects to work on every other weekend. His graduation wouldn't be until a few weeks after our son's due date. But I knew that he had been wanting to grow his skills for some time, and I thought if not now, then when? Yes, I would eat dinner alone most nights, pack lunch *and* dinner, and make weekend plans and go to appointments without Luis. Yet, Luis would be doing this not only for himself but for our family, and I knew what my part was—it was to take care of us, and I happily took on that challenge.

Luis and I understood that a late pregnancy loss was still possible, but with such a healthy, practically textbook pregnancy, we didn't worry too much. Instead, we "worried" about things most first-time parents worry about, like getting the nursery together, finding the safest car seat, and taking the prenatal classes. I even recall telling a friend that I knew that it was a possibility that I could have a stillbirth or that something could happen after he was born, but all I could do was focus on what was within my control. I couldn't tell the future and could only focus on the present. In a way, I felt a sense of peace in doing what I could control and letting the rest go. I never felt such a peace in my life. Looking back, I believe that Massimo gave me this gift—this clarity of mind that continues to help pull me out from the depths of intense guilt and sorrow in my grief, and from debilitating fear and anxiety during my subsequent pregnancy.

Something we delighted in was wondering about his personality. Our first son was due in the year of the Fire Rooster. It became somewhat of a nickname, and even some of our friends joined in the fun. We kept his name a secret, so he became known as our Fire Rooster. Would he be energetic? A handful? Super social? This big personality felt so right. It fit the plaque a friend gave to us at our shower with the inscription, "Let him sleep, for when he wakes he will move mountains." When our childbirth class leader asked us to bring in a focal point to help us breathe through the contractions for our hopefully unmedicated natural birth, we chose this plaque. Most couples brought in an ultrasound photo, but we wanted this plaque because it represented our hopes and dreams for Massimo.

Occasionally, the haunting memory of how we discussed our little Fire Rooster's possible traits as we waited at labor and delivery on that wretched Friday visits me. I had heard his heartbeat and tracked his movements in my nonstress test two days earlier. At that appointment, I had my membranes swept, as I was already one centimeter dilated. I felt him move the day after the appointment and excitedly walked around my neighborhood and bounced on my birthing ball. That Friday night I awoke, as I usually do, to use the toilet. However, I thought I didn't feel him move as much that evening, so I ate something. I sat in the rocking chair and sang, "Sleep Baby Sleep," to him. I swear I felt him move, enough for me to return to sleep.

The next morning, I didn't feel him move after breakfast. I called my midwife's office, and they told me to lie on my left side, drink ice water, and eat something. We headed to labor and delivery when he continued to not respond. Even though I was going in because of reduced movements at forty-one weeks, we spoke with excitement and hope, not knowing that our world was about to crumble. Thinking back, I believe he was already gone that Friday morning.

Shock engulfed me as I realized that I would still need to deliver him. I don't know how or when, but I remember thinking, I have to do this— welcoming our son into this world was what we'd been preparing for, and it would be one of the last things we could do for him.

As the fierce fire of the sun arose in the sky that Saturday morning, our son was born still.

We named him Massimo Loi Cabrera.

Massimo, an Italian name, meaning the greatest; Loi, a Vietnamese name, after my father; and Cabrera, to carry the Dominican family name.

Yes, great sorrow was in that delivery room, but the overwhelming feelings were joy and pride. We stared at him in awe, our beautiful baby boy, our firstborn. On his birthday, I finally understood what it was like to experience all of the beauty and tragedy that life has to offer. What an intimate, holy, and brutal experience to share with my husband. All of it and all that is to come—every thought, feeling, and experience in the messy world of grief—are rooted in love. People say there are no words, but that is the only word, Love.

I continue to learn much from Massimo. Several months after the fog of the raw grief started to fade, I realized that I didn't know how I was going to navigate this new world of grief and, frankly, my life going forward, but I vowed that I would not let his death destroy me or my marriage. That would not be a part of my son's legacy. Instead, I wanted to live brightly for Massimo. If he could live so fearlessly in his short life, so could I. He has awoken me and I will move mountains.

The Ritual

Rona Fernandez

Once a week, I buy her flowers. Her colors are purple and pink, so I pick blush-colored baby roses, neon Gerber daisies, white lilies with fuchsia centers, violet-blue irises. And foliage to round out the arrangement: glossy camellia leaves, gray-toned eucalyptus, feathery green ferns. I have my favorite spots to buy the flowers—the grocery store in our neighborhood, the farmer's market when it's the right season. I avoid the cheap flowers at the supermarket that I know will die within a day or two; those aren't good enough for this. A few times a year, a thoughtful friend will drop off flowers from her garden, usually on the more difficult days. But I don't expect anyone else to take this task on. This is my job as her mother, though I wish it wasn't.

This is how I mother my child.

* * *

My daughter's name is Naima Kali—like the Coltrane song, and the Hindu goddess of creation. She was born on March 25, 2011, her due date. The nurses said this was a rare thing. But I didn't schedule her birth—it was too sacred an event to coordinate around my common needs. Still, my daughter came right on time, and I birthed her the old-fashioned way, took no drugs to shield me from the intensity and immensity of labor. I wanted to be fully present during the birth of my first child, wanted to feel it all—pain, ecstasy, fatigue, joy, overwhelm, all.

The contractions started in earnest the night before she was born, a drizzly Bay Area spring evening, cool and quiet. They were waves of energy that started in my full womb, rocking me from inside out, drawing guttural moans from a deep, primal place inside me. People stared at me, wide-eyed, as I walked past them in the hospital lobby, leaning heavily on my husband Henry's arm as we made our way to the maternity ward. I felt powerful and vulnerable at the same time, sensing that my body was fully in control, that my mind would need to surrender and let my body do this job that it had been created for.

Through the night, the contractions fatigued me as they stretched and opened my womb, my eyelids becoming so heavy that the biggest worry became whether I could stay awake until the end. I kept trying to nap, thinking the *real labor* was still coming, not knowing that I was in the midst of it, that this was it.

Then finally, after twelve hours of active labor and more than three hours of pushing, she arrived.

I heard my Naima before I ever saw her, for she screamed aloud as she emerged from my body, announcing herself, lungs filling with air, already demanding attention. Henry and our midwife caught her as she was born. As they placed her on my chest, I chanted, shouting, "My baby! My baby!"

Relief and gratitude and love commingled in a deep wave of emotion as my body released her. She was pink, perfect, her rounded, moist head lifted slightly as she was placed on top of me, her eyes—double-lidded, caramel brown, and beautiful, just like my husband's—were already open, and she stared *straight at me*. Naima had an intensity even at birth that will always stay with me.

Bonding is a shallow way to describe what happened between my daughter and me at that moment. Our eyes met for that first time and—*bam*—that was it. She was mine, I was hers, we were connected immutably from that moment on. I knew then that I would do anything to keep her safe, happy.

Soon, Naima was latched onto my breast, her dark-pink mouth strong and voracious. Henry and I gazed down at her in awe, both feeling something that the word *love* only scratches the surface of. There is a photo of the three of us at this moment, my dark hair damp with sweat, Henry's dark eyes shining with pride, tiny Naima bundled in a white, pink, and blue blanket in my arms. Our little, perfect, new family.

* * *

I often arrange the flowers during a moment of quiet, when I'm home, alone. It's a silent prayer that I shape with my hands, as I carefully place each blossom and stem in a water-filled vase.

This is how I mother my daughter now, but I wish that I could mother her in other, more normal ways. Wish that I could teach her how to tie her shoes or put her clothes on right side out, wish that I could make tiny pencil marks on the wall in her bedroom to show how much she's grown each year. Wish that I could cook her favorite food for her—maybe it would have been pizza, or lumpia, or noodles—or watch my husband teach her how to ride a bike. Wish that I could hear her cry *Mommy* after falling off the jungle gym at the park or comfort her when she has a fever.

These are the precious moments that most parents take for granted: the small, everyday witnessings of life as their child grows and changes. I wish I could have all these things.

But I can't. Because my daughter, my first and only born, my Naima, is not here. She is dead.

Naima does not have a grave. My husband and I could not bear the thought of her body going into the cold ground alone. So, her ashes sit in a silver urn on our mantle, so that we will never be completely without her. The urn has three blue birds etched deeply into its surface, flying free and wild. I like to think that the birds represent the three of us—mother, father, child—and that someday we will see each other again and fly away together into the ether.

This is my weekly ritual—flowers, silence, remembrance. It gives me some comfort. I place the pink and purple flowers in a vase, pray that my daughter feels the love that her father and I have for her, pray that she is free and in bliss somewhere, flying high like the birds on the small, silver urn that holds her ashes, pray that she knows how grateful we are for her, even now.

This is how I mother my child.

* * *

The three of us spent all of our time together in the first six weeks of Naima's life, getting to know each other, following her cues and cries and needs, learning this new rhythm of life as a family, learning how to love in this new, dizzying, and delightful way.

Though she slept well at night—an unexpected blessing—Naima was averse to daytime naps. Instead, she wanted to nurse almost constantly (and developed famously chubby cheeks as a result; one friend joked that they looked like they had round *siopao* buns stuffed into them) and cried if we put her down for more than a couple minutes when she was awake. Naima's newborn cry was piercing and demanding, and all the more shocking since she was so tiny—she weighed not quite six pounds at birth. Our hearts would never let her wail for long, so we held Naima for most of her waking hours in those early weeks, as we read and watched lots of television, our arms developing muscles and stamina we hadn't known they could. Like many things about parenthood, you push yourself beyond what you think you can do, and are constantly surprised by what you are capable of enduring.

Naima was not quite one month old when Henry had to meet with our accountant to get our taxes done. I still didn't want to bring her to too many new places for fear of germs and viruses, but I longed to get out of the house for fresh air, so we decided that Henry would drop me and the baby off at the Rose Garden for our first-ever walk without Daddy, while he met with our accountant. I was excited, couldn't wait to be a mom in public, pushing around my baby in her cute, gray-and-orange stroller.

At the park, Henry kissed us goodbye and left as I began to push Naima in her stroller, gratefully inhaling the crisp springtime air against my face. But my smile didn't last long, because it soon became clear that Naima did not like being in her stroller *at all*. She wailed nonstop, her cry carrying on the breeze like an alarm. I took her out and nursed her, standing up in the middle of the Rose Garden, a bit embarrassed, hoping that she would fall asleep so we could continue our walk. Because isn't that what one is supposed to do with newborns? Have pleasant walks in the park with them as they snooze innocently?

But Naima had other plans. Every time I put her down in her stroller, she just cried and cried until I picked her up again. I did this at least half a dozen times, but it didn't work, and I couldn't just let her cry, knowing that her cry meant *I need something* and that I, as her mother, needed to figure out what that something was and give it to her, whatever it was. So I gave in to the tremendous force of will of my three-week-old baby and sat on a park bench and nursed her, the abandoned stroller nearby. I felt frustrated and exhausted—I had failed at my first real attempt at a public display of contented new motherhood.

My frustration soon dissipated, however, when I looked down at Naima in my arms. She was quiet now, lying snugly against my body, almond-shaped eyes closed, her mouth fastened to my breast, cheeks pulsing with the instinctive effort of nursing contentedly. In giving up and giving in to my daughter, I had won a small victory, the kind that all new mothers eventually come to know and understand and appreciate: a happy, satisfied baby.

And in the end, that was all that really mattered.

* * *

When I first tell people about my daughter, I usually say that she *passed away*. But that's a euphemism, isn't it? A way to soften the jagged edges of the truth: that my daughter, my Naima, my first- and only-born child, is dead.

In response, people say trite, canned things.

She'll always be with you. She lives on in your heart. Don't worry, you'll have another baby or *She's an angel watching over you now.*

These are often people who have living children, parents who can wrap their arms around their child or give them a kiss on the cheek, who don't have to wonder what their child would have looked like at two, twelve, or twenty-five years old.

I can count on two hands the number of times that I told people about my daughter who simply replied, "I'm so sorry." Can count even fewer times that they ask what her name is or if I want to show them a picture. Sometimes they say nothing at all, just continue on as if I haven't just revealed the most painful truth of my life to them, as if I've just told them something obvious, like *The Earth is round*.

For better or worse, I've become accustomed to these silent responses. If I'm feeling particularly emotional that day, I will go somewhere quiet and cry, alone. Crying is a normal part of life now, something I've learned to accept, even embrace. I can cry while doing all sorts of things: cooking, driving, walking down the street, taking a shower, petting my dog, writing. Crying is necessary now and often comforting, like arranging the flowers.

I place the flowers in a clear crystal vase next to her urn, besides which is a favorite picture of Naima—her eyes, clear-seeing and pure, stare straight at me, her cheeks plump and flush and full of life, a serious baby, a perfect baby. Half the time, the image makes me smile, the other half, it makes me weep.

* * *

I searched and searched for the right day care to bring my daughter to once she turned three months old. I took comfort in knowing it would be for just two days a week—the rest of the week she was with me, or her Daddy, or both of us. I had planned it this way and could work at home sometimes, so that I could spend as much time with our daughter as possible.

Of course, I would have preferred to keep her home with me, to have a nanny who could attend to us both whenever I needed to go anywhere, but we couldn't afford it, and also, it felt selfish. I wanted Naima to be around other children, to hear other little ones' laughter and talking and singing and crying, to be around the special delight and playfulness and crankiness that only children can exhibit. It was how I was raised, and my young childhood had been the happiest time of my life.

I found a place where a friend had had her baby for three years, from infancy through toddlerhood. It was less than two miles from our home, easy to get to, and located in a quiet, diverse, safe, tree-lined Oakland neighborhood. It felt like the right place, run by an older, Christian immigrant couple—Mr. and Mrs. Kim—who clearly cherished all the children they cared for.

Though I was nervous and sad to drop her off on her first day, Naima took to the day care immediately. There were a few other children, ages nine months to four years old, at the day care, and I knew Naima would not feel lonely, even if she missed me. Later that day, when I picked her up and brought her home, I noticed Naima lying in her playpen making sounds I had never heard her make before, little baby-talk sounds that I attributed to the lively, playful environment at the Kims'. This made me smile.

On a warm summer day in late July, I took Naima to her four-month checkup. The kind doctor, whom I had picked specifically out of the Kaiser directory after researching all the family doctors, examined Naima carefully, questioned me thoroughly, and was gentle with my baby. She pronounced Naima "perfect" and sent us on our way.

* * *

That day. August third. What shall I tell you about it? Do you really want to know?

I could tell you that it was a beautiful, perfect summer day, that I had no idea that my happy family was going to be destroyed. About how my husband and I had dropped her off that morning together, which was rare, because I was giving him a ride to the train station before a work meeting I had downtown. I could tell you that I knew something was wrong when I checked my phone—which had been on silent because of my work meeting—and saw that the babysitter had called not once but twice. When I called back on their landline, it was busy. Panic closed my throat.

Don't let anything be wrong, please.

I could tell you how I dialed their cell phone next, about how Mr. Kim answered the phone with the clipped words, *The baby stopped breathing.* I could tell you how I screamed and ran out of the house, how I don't even remember if I had my purse or anything but the car keys in my hand. I drove to the day care and almost hit several cars, chanting *Hold on, baby, wait for Mommy, Mommy's coming,* as if my daughter could hear me, as if my words could make a difference. I was her Mommy, couldn't I make everything better? I could tell you how I somehow believed that once I got there, she would start breathing again and everything would be okay.

I could tell you how just writing these words now makes me burst into tears, makes me lose my breath. I could tell you about how I called 911 as I drove, how I felt a strange, slight sliver of relief when I pulled up in front of the day care and saw an ambulance and firetruck and police truck there.

She has to be okay.

I could tell you how I screamed when I saw my daughter's tiny body laid out on the living-room coffee table at the day care, how the fire fighters pumped her tiny chest, and I shouted, *I'm right here, baby, Mommy's right here,* and how they wouldn't let me near her. I sobbed, trying to get the policeman whose brawny arm kept me from charging toward my daughter—*They need space to work on her*—to look me in the eye, needing reassurance that Naima was going to be okay. He wouldn't look at me.

I could tell you how I felt utterly useless, how I finally called my husband because there was nothing they would let me, her mother, do. Later, he would tell me that I was crying, he couldn't understand what I was saying. By the time I was able to explain what was going on, the paramedics were taking Naima away to Children's Hospital. The firemen pulled me toward their truck to drive me there. I begged to go with her in the ambulance, but they wouldn't let me. I just wanted to be near my baby, I knew she would wake up for Mommy. She always woke up for Mommy.

I could tell you about how my husband and I stood outside the emergency room door, how I prayed more prayers in those five minutes of waiting than I had ever prayed in my life. I could tell you how my husband cursed when he saw, how I screamed when they told me, how I had to be held up so that I wouldn't collapse to the floor, how everything after that moment was a blur of tears and agony—not just for days or weeks but for months.

I could tell you more, of course, but it's just too hard.

What I will tell you is that Naima died in her sleep at day care. They call it sudden infant death syndrome, or SIDS, which just means that they don't really know what happened. They told us there was nothing we could have done, no way we could have saved her. I still don't understand how that could be. I'm her mother, there must have been something I did wrong, something I missed.

* * *

It happens less frequently now, but I still have those doubting moments, the moments when I blame myself for her death. *Should I have taken her with me to work that day? Should I not have had the wine at my sister's wedding that weekend? Should I have not listened to the doctor when they told me to feed her formula as a newborn, to clear her jaundice? Should I have? Should I?*

This is how I mother my child.

Some weeks, I get so busy that I can't find the time for my little ritual, my days filled with mundane tasks—work deadlines, cooking or cleaning, running errands. Sometimes I let the flowers sit too long in the holding vase that I put them in after I bring them home from the store. After a few days they start to wither—some of the petals fall off, the pinks and purples begin to fade. I feel guilty when this happens, as if I've forgotten her, having fallen down on my one, simple task now that she's gone.

I try to remember that letting the flowers sit out a few days doesn't mean that I love her any less. I remind myself that if Naima were still here, I would probably feel guilty instead about yelling at her in a moment of frustration, or about forgetting what she wanted for Christmas, or about being late to pick her up from kindergarten.

But that's not my reality. What I have instead are wilted flowers and tears.

I try to be gentle with myself in these moments, remind myself that these things happen. It's not easy being the mother of a dead child. In fact, it may be the hardest kind of mothering there is.

This is how I mother my child: Once a week, I buy flowers for her. I create a bouquet of purples and pinks and greens. I put it next to her urn. I pray for her, miss her, remember her, and love her.

Always, always love her.

The Night Parade

Jami Nakamura Lin

April 2018. This is an ongoing tale. The ending is still uncertain. Daily I examine the toilet paper every time I wipe, nightly I read my underwear like tea leaves, searching for the rust that means ruin. I try to talk myself down: this is okay, and this is okay, and today, everything is okay. Once in a while I believe the story I tell.

My pregnancies—the one I lost and the one that is ongoing, the one that is *to be determined*—I think about in fragments, and thus my retelling is fragmented. Maybe this is a convenient excuse, an easy out to explain away the lack of narrative cohesion, to sidestep that niggling issue that my advisor called the *so what* of the essay.

I lost a baby. *So what?* As of today, I am having another one. *So what?*

I

September 2017. These days I can't stop thinking about origins. Maybe it's the time of year: autumn in Chicago, the briefest of seasons. Because our schedule revolves heavily around my husband Aaron's academic calendar, September is always the true start of the year, whereas January means just a turn of the calendar page. Or maybe it's because my small group is reading through the book of Genesis, which opens: *In the beginning . . .*

But most likely it's because this is the month I go to the doctor to have my intrauterine device removed. Next month, Aaron and I are "going to start to try," a vague, euphemistic phrase that piles beginning upon beginning.

Originally (*in the beginning*) we had planned on waiting until the following January to take out my IUD. But then, over the summer, my father is diagnosed with terminal cancer. My generous, loving father who, dopey on drugs in the hospital, tells me how much he wants grandchildren. He wants to be called *Agon,* the Taiwanese word for grandpa, the word we used for his own father, who died when I was young.

So Aaron and I decide to start trying a little earlier. I cannot think about the timeline, about where my father will be in nine months. Even as I type this it hurts. So this is enough.

* * *

Though the majority of the tales in Genesis revolve around the men— Adam and his rib, Noah and his ark, Abraham and his covenant, Joseph and his dreams—I follow the matriarchs. What I understand is their longing. What I understand is their need.

For example. Abraham's wife, Sarah, who had yearned for a child for years, whose childlessness had brought her so much anguish, was ninety when God told her she would finally—*finally!*—bear a son. She laughed in God's face.

Then the Lord said to Abraham, "Why did Sarah laugh and say, 'Will I really have a child, now that I am old?' Is anything too hard for the Lord? . . ."

Sarah was afraid, so she lied and said, "I did not laugh."

But he said, "Yes, you did laugh."

What I understand is their disbelief that God would give them a good thing.

* * *

I whip myself into a frenzy of action. I meet with a certified nurse-midwife to make sure that my body is all ready to go in October. I make a plan with my psychiatrist about how we will taper off my bipolar medications once I'm pregnant. I talk to my therapist about all these fears, and we plot soothing strategies and coping mechanisms.

But for every minute I spend praying or trying to calm myself, I spend sixty perusing the baby boards, the websites and forums dedicated to assisting women through their pregnancies. While the articles and blog posts are genuinely helpful, the message boards—the meat and potatoes of these sites—serve only to feed my anxiety. There's a post by a vetted medical professional that tells me that spotting and cramping in early pregnancy can be completely normal; there are also thousands of excruciatingly detailed posts by women for whom spotting was the first sign of the end. This is the problem with the Internet Age: the information is endless, and endlessly terrifying.

From the boards I learn about "symptom spotting"—tracking your pregnancy symptoms (or lack thereof) during the "2ww"—the two-week wait between when you ovulate and when you can take a pregnancy test. Boobs sore? Nauseous? Overly hungry? Not hungry at all? These are all "symptoms" that these women, many of them who have experienced repeat pregnancy loss, many who have struggled with infertility, look for. Most of the women will admit up front that what they are doing is illogical, that the signs don't *really* mean anything at this point. And yet. Here they are. Here I am.

It's ten in the morning and I'm on the boards. It's midnight and I'm on the boards. It's the only place where others' anxiety matches my own. People in my own life, my husband, for example, don't understand why I am so nervous. I have not experienced any loss or pregnancy-related struggle of my own. But my family, I try to explain. But my genes. But my bipolar disorder.

I know my addiction to these boards is unhealthy. And yet. On the boards, the women understand without any explanation. They don't try to dissuade you from your irrational thoughts. They don't try to spew facts at you. Instead, they say, *Hugs, mama.* They say, *I know. It's so hard.* They know the fear that waits and watches, that breathes every time you take a breath.

* * *

I come from a people who birth with difficulty. The women in my family fought for the children they had. My mother, with her three daughters, probably had the "easiest" time of all; still we grew up with a rose bush in our garden to commemorate the child she lost after me.

My aunts on both my Japanese and Taiwanese sides have struggled. Miscarriage, infertility, infant loss. Growing up, what I took away from this was that wanting a baby in no way guarantees getting a baby. I was young. I did not know the statistics. What I knew was what was in front of me: pregnancy is hard, infertility common, miscarriages frequent. What I knew was my aunt and uncle praying at night with my cousin for years: *and please bring him a little baby brother.*

They say that many women are uninformed about how common miscarriage is. I had the opposite problem. I thought, for me, with my lineage, it would be the default.

And yet: everyone in my family has at least one child. There is that.

* * *

October 2017. Our first month trying. During the two-week wait, I am certain I am pregnant. I write in my journal that I just *feel* different. *I can't tell anyone because they'd think I'm crazy,* I write. *But I'm writing it here, first, as proof.* I take a test much too early and wait for the second line to show up. It doesn't. Next day, same routine, same result. This goes on for three or four days until I start to spot.

I hope that it's just implantation bleeding—when the embryo attaches to your lining, it can cause blood that some mistake for a period—but the next day and its river of red proves to me otherwise. I am sad in a way my husband doesn't understand, a sadness that, later on, will seem so inconsequential.

*   *   *

November 2017. Our second month of trying. Though I am "temping" (taking my temperature with my basal thermometer every day to track my thermal shifts throughout my cycle) and using OPKs (ovulation predictor kits—strips that look like pregnancy tests that you pee on to determine when you're ovulating), I am sure I didn't time our sex correctly and that we're out for this month. Unlike last month, when I started peeing on a stick a week before my period was supposed to come, this month I don't think about it at all until I realize my period is late.

Two blazing lines right away.

Um, I call from the bathroom, opening the door with my foot. We're pregnant.

My husband runs over and looks at the stick I hold up in two hands like an offering. My pants and underwear still at my ankles.

Hurray! he says. Can we not have a gender reveal party?

My parents are overjoyed with the news.

When my father speaks of his friends from my Japanese-American church—whose parents were friends with my grandparents, whose children are my own friends—he talks about how much they love their grandchildren, and says they can't have all the fun. He is so excited for us. When he sees two toddlers, cousins, poke their heads above a pew in front of us, he leans over and whispers, I want one of those.

My mother's cousin texts me: *You think it's your baby, but it's all of ours.* She's only partially joking. I am the oldest in my generation on both sides of the family, and they are all deeply invested in the life growing in my womb. While others might find this claustrophobic, our Asian sense of family and community is what gives me peace when I think about raising our child. We will not be alone.

* * *

December 2017. I have my first ultrasound. We see our baby, which looks like a gray blob. The crown-to-rump length marks it at eight weeks, one day. I take a picture of the sonogram with my phone and send it to all our family and close friends. Aaron and I go to Stan's Donuts afterwards to celebrate. I order three for myself: a cruller, a Boston creme, an apple fritter. I'm pregnant. We're pregnant.

The ultrasound is on Tuesday. The following Sunday I start spotting. I am very worried, but I try to tamp it down: spotting in pregnancy can be normal, I tell myself. There's no cramping. I'm not filling a pad. I keep my panic in check.

Three days later, when I'm still spotting, I message my midwife. The next morning, she emails me that it might be nothing, but I can come in for an ultrasound just to check things out. She has an appointment available at ten. Or, she says, I can wait a little longer to see what happens.

I am bad at waiting.

I call her office and take the ten o'clock appointment. It is 9:25. If I leave now, I'll barely make it. I drive, frenzied, sobbing from my gut. Please, please, I pray as traffic stalls along Lake Shore Drive, please let the baby be alive, please let me get there in time. I call my mother, who says she will drive in from the suburbs to meet me.

I am late, but the midwife isn't ready for me anyway. I pee in a cup, and it is filled with webby red strands that look like those I know. Finally, I am led into a room. My mother gets there just as the midwife takes the ultrasound wand out.

Her silence is everything. I am supposed to be almost ten weeks. The baby is measuring eight weeks, four days.

Another doctor comes in. She confirms that there is no heartbeat, no blood flow to the baby.

I'm so sorry, I tell my mother, who weeps harder than me. I cry too, but not hard, not like in the car, when I still didn't know. Now I know.

I was right, I think. I knew that this would be the way it ended.

* * *

Because I am so far along, the midwife recommends a D&C. My husband takes off work, and we go to the hospital the next day. We wait around for many hours. It is all very simple. The worst part about it is when the nurse can't find my vein for the IV. I am put under. They take everything dead out of me. I wake up, and my husband and I get Shake Shack. We take a photo and send it to my family to show them I am okay.

I feel that I have let my entire family down. I cannot bear to talk to them about it. My mother disseminates the news. When my grandparents call, when my aunt leaves a message, I do not pick up.

There is also a sense of relief: that what I had expected would happen this whole time had actually happened, and now it is over.

* * *

I read a lot of essays and blog posts about miscarriage after my experience—all of them by white women of privilege. I suppose that they are the ones who have platforms and time to blog. The blog posts especially are so aesthetically pleasing—littered with photographs of the bloggers, beautifully styled, looking into the distance, or rocking in a wicker chair on a porch with the sun setting behind them—that I cannot stomach it. All the comments talk about how brave they are.

One of the problems is that these blog posts are one-offs, a one-time intimate look on what is usually a lifestyle blog. The rest of the posts—before and after—are again about how to refurbish your barn door, how to water your succulents. What I can understand better are the blogs set up specifically for women going through infertility, but I am not going through infertility. But I identify with the heaviness present in all their posts, even the ones about the rest of their daily lives, because infertility is a weight you carry around constantly. Miscarriage is often treated like an event that happens and is over.

The thing is: luckily, miscarriage is often just an event, not a lifestyle. It *is* over, and women go on to have many children.

How to hold both these ideas in your hand?

The women writing about miscarriage don't look like me. They don't sound like me. There is nothing that *resonates*. I want a quote that I can watercolor in my sadness and put on my wall.

* * *

January 2018. I begin this essay on January 1, two weeks after my D&C, still reeling from our loss. And yet in that pain there is also stillness. There are no unknown quantities. The thing I was most afraid of has happened.

My midwife tells me to wait until I get my period again before trying again. So we wait. For the first time in our marriage, we use condoms. Seeing the box sitting on my husband's bedside table is depressing. Having sex with the condom on is depressing. To prevent the thing we most want.

Finally, I find a quote worthy of watercoloring, only it's not in an essay about miscarriage, and it's not about miscarriage at all. In Hanya Yanagihara's *A Little Life,* a father ruminates about the aftermath of his child's death:

But here's what no one says—when it's your child, a part of you, a very tiny but nonetheless unignorable part of you, also feels relief. Because finally, the moment you have been expecting, been dreading, been preparing yourself for since the day you became a parent, has come.

Ah, you tell yourself, it's arrived. Here it is.

And after that, you have nothing to fear again.

Though I wouldn't compare my first-term pregnancy loss with the loss of the character's grown son, this quote sums up what I feel. I am devastated, yes, and I had expected to be devastated.

II

I wait for forty days before I bleed—the first benchmark. I start tracking my temperature again. I wait another three weeks until I reach my fertile window, the days around ovulation. Aaron and I have a lot of sex. I wait another two weeks.

February 2018. I tell Aaron I won't take a pregnancy test until I miss my period. That's a good idea, he says. It *is* a good idea but an unachievable one. I test six days before I'm supposed to miss my period.

I am pregnant. Again. For about one second I am elated. I know we are lucky, blessed. I know—now that I am armed with statistics, too many to handle—how often women have to wait an unspeakably long time for what in trying-to-conceive parlance are called *rainbow babies,* the babies that come after the storm of miscarriage, stillbirth, or infant loss.

The thing about fear: how insidious it is. How a drop of fear can taint a whole bucket of happiness.

What they didn't tell me to expect when I was expecting again: how it feels worse in some ways than those weeks after the miscarriage, when I wasn't yet pregnant. Then I was afraid in the abstract. Now that I am again *with child,* I carry the fear too, deep in my belly.

You see, when a good thing has been taken from you, it is hard to believe that you will be able to hold it in your hands.

Do not be anxious about anything, the Bible says, *but in prayer and petition, in every situation, with Thanksgiving, present your requests to God.*

I present my requests. And still I am afraid. If I were stronger, I think, if I had more faith.

* * *

March 2018. My psychiatrist and I work out a plan to taper off of my medications again. After I miscarried, I went back on, and so now I have to wean off. Since the first time went so well, I am not expecting any problems.

During the first pregnancy I thought I had been afraid. Now I know what it is to be afraid, and I feel it in my body and my mind. I cannot talk about the pregnancy without qualifying it: *if, if.*

My fear somatized looks like extreme agitation. I'd had these symptoms as a teenager, before being diagnosed with bipolar, but in the decade since, I've forgotten what it's like: a flailing. A thrashing. Rolling around on the floor, on the bed, pulling at my hair, scratching at my skin. I call my psychiatrist, who adjusts my dosing schedule so I wean more slowly.

I cannot concentrate. This is a blend of being in my first trimester, when every woman is probably some level of discombobulated, and being off my medications. I am tired. I am writing in simple sentences, in separate chunks, hoping that they will come together. I am too tired for subordinate clauses and complex syntax, too tired to focus on more than one paragraph at a time.

To people who ask how I am doing, I refer to my frenzies as psychomotor agitation. I use the word my psychiatrist uses: *akathisia.* It's too ludicrous to try to explain what this feels like. What it looks like is a toddler throwing a tantrum. A twenty-eight-year-old woman racing to the recycling container in the kitchen and fishing out the largest Amazon Prime boxes, then ripping each one into pieces. Paper is not satisfying—it succumbs to my will too easily. My therapist recommends ripping up a phone book, but who has a phone book anymore? The boxes are hard to tear into but not impossible. It takes exertion. Ripping releases my energy, though not my fear.

My husband tucks me under my twenty-pound weighted blanket, climbs straight on top of me, curving his spine up so he won't put pressure on my belly—he is always concerned about smushing the baby, no matter what I tell him—grabs me with his arms and legs and rocks me back and forth.

Squeeze me as hard as you can, I tell him. Harder than that. Harder. Later in life I discovered, with my therapist's help, that the coping skills and methods used for people on the autism spectrum also help me when I'm spiraling. Weight, pressure, motion: these often, but not always, stop the flailing.

When the coping skills don't work, I rage, stomp around the house, throw my phone. The episodes last "only" fifteen minutes or so, but that quarter of an hour feels like nights. My poor husband. Afterwards, a half an hour, an hour of crying, of me apologizing, *I'm sorry, I'm so sorry, what grown woman, what kind of grown woman*—

* * *

As I get further into Genesis, I have to come to grips with the truth. I am not like the matriarchs of the Bible. The women in Genesis give me hope, but I do not see my face in their faces: waiting, obedient. I see my face in the woodblock prints of the *yokai* I find in my research on Japanese mythology, the legendary supernatural spirits and creatures and demons.

During the summer, the stories go, they journey through the streets of Japan in a long procession. Anyone who has the bad luck to stumble upon the *yokai* will be "spirited away." This is called the Night Parade of One Hundred Demons.

Some of these *yokai* are ghosts, and some of these ghosts are women, and some of these women look more like me than not. Pale and haggard, always with long, black hair, bedraggled and knotted, an external representation of the roiling inside them.

For these formerly human women are in turmoil, which prevents them from crossing peacefully into the afterlife. Perhaps someone had committed a crime against them. Perhaps they had a score to settle. Perhaps they'd suffered a loss. For whatever reason, they could not let go. Instead they remain on earth, haunting others, until whatever strong emotion tethers them to this physical plane is released. They need absolution, and until they receive it, they remain as "faint spirits," haunting the world during the hour of the ox (one to three in the morning), when the fabric between the living and the dead is the most permeable.

These are the women I think about when I can't sleep. These women who have lost something.

* * *

What does it mean to trust I write in my journal. I agonize that I cannot let go of my fear, and I am frustrated that the things that soothe me are the tangible. Heartbeat, Doppler, ultrasound. *But faith is being sure of what you hope for, and certain of what you do not see.* But I like seeing.

I carry the fear like the baby's invisible twin, or more like a subchorionic hematoma—a condition some pregnant women face, when a pocket of blood forms in the uterus. Sometimes the hematoma gets smaller over time, and everything is fine. In some cases, it can cause a miscarriage. If you see this on your ultrasound, it's often just a waiting game.

I know that expecting the worst is not an effective weapon against calamity, but it seems at times to be all that I have—a balm that poisons.

When I have my ultrasound, the technician doesn't tell me what I desperately want to know: that everything is okay. It is seven thirty at night; the hospital is empty. We are in a large, dimly lit room, barren but for the table for me to lie on and the ultrasound equipment. She takes so many photos, so many more than at my first ultrasound, that I feel certain something is wrong.

You'll have to wait until your midwife calls you for your results, she says.

She was so chilly! I complain to my husband after. She didn't tell us anything, I'm sure there's a problem.

He tells me he didn't notice anything strange in her manner. But he wouldn't; he's not on high alert.

I examine the photograph of our ultrasound and tried to imagine all the potential problems. Please, I prayed, please let it only be a subchorionic hematoma. In that case I still had a chance. The other option, I felt, was that there was something wrong with the baby itself. A hematoma I could handle.

Instead nothing was wrong. I did not think of this as a real possibility.

* * *

When Rachel saw that she was not bearing Jacob any children, she became jealous of her sister. So she said to Jacob, "Give me children, or I'll die!"

Jacob became angry with her and said, "Am I in the place of God, who has kept you from having children?"

Then she said, "Here is Bilhah, my servant. Sleep with her so that she can bear children for me and I too can build a family through her."

We make our own contingency plans.

* * *

April 2018: My nausea is going away, I tell Aaron. Good! He says. Once I throw up in front of him and my sister and her boyfriend while we are all in the car together. We don't have a bag, so my sister, an illustrator, yanks one of her art prints from its flimsy cellophane envelope. Aaron holds it for me while I gag and puke, and then he holds it gingerly, with his finger and thumb, while I drive home.

The car fogged up like in that scene with the velociraptors in *Jurassic Park,* Aaron recounts to my parents.

You have a good husband my parents tell me again. I know.

It makes me nervous, I tell him. That I'm feeling better.

I know this is normal, that at this stage the placenta starts taking over, and the pregnancy symptoms wane. I am relieved to not be nauseous all the time, and yet in the absence of it I do not find peace but fear. I had no symptoms with my first pregnancy, and that one ended. Some studies have shown a correlation between lack of morning sickness and miscarriage.

Jami, my husband says, with the mix of love and exasperation so common to marriage, there is no pleasing you.

* * *

April 2018: My father's CT scan shows eight new tumors. We are not sure if we can go on our trip to Taiwan this summer.

On the plus side, he tells me—when I call him just to hear his voice, because the only thing that can calm me when I hear such news is his voice because his voice means he is here and he is alive—on the plus side, if I get the surgery in the summer, it means I'll *definitely* be out by November, and we won't be in the hospital at the same time!

That had been one of his worries, that he would be recuperating from his operation at his hospital in the suburbs at the same time I was delivering in the city. That he wouldn't be able to be there for my birth.

My parents speak about the baby like it is a given. *When* you have the baby. It is so hard for me to believe that we will take home a baby and it will be fine, though this is the most statistically likely scenario. After everything with my father, I expect the worst in all situations.

I worry about all my worry. It's bad for the baby, the Internet tells me. Stress can lead to miscarriage. So I talk to the baby. I sing to it. When I hear the heartbeat at my ten-week appointment, I begin, slowly, to believe. I create a Pinterest board of all the crafts I want to make for the nursery. I start knitting a Totoro stuffed animal.

* * *

We announce our pregnancy at twelve weeks exactly. The night before, curled in bed on my left side (the better for the baby to receive blood flow), I invent different drafts of status updates. I want to talk about my miscarriage, but it seems wrong to mention that in the same breath as a new baby. I worry that people will not know how to respond, that they will feel compelled to temper their happiness the way mine is tempered.

What I want to say: *Today we are twelve weeks. After everything, getting to this point seems like—is—a miracle.* What I say: *The Center for Jewish-Japanese Relations* [my husband's and my pet name for our household] *is premiering its best project yet!*

What I want to say: *A lot of fear. A lot of trepidation. And yet: a lot of prayer and a lot of joy.* What I say: two star-eyes emoji, two puke-face emoji.

After posting this truth-but-not-the-whole-truth announcement, I worry about how this will affect an old college friend who posts honestly about how hard it is to see pregnancy announcements after her own infertility and pregnancy loss. (And how many women like her yet invisible.)

Among all the likes and congratulatory messages, her comment—an image of a rainbow, with no text—stands out to me the most. What grace.

What my post says: *Things are great!* What I want to say: *Thus far.*

145

* * *

Another fear: who am I to speak of this sorrow, when so many other women have seen so much more? My relative luck is most salient to me on the motherhood forums where I stew in my anxiety and lurk the day away. On these baby boards, you have the option of adding a signature, which works the same way as email signatures: the text pops up every time you post. Only instead of listing a phone number and address, as you would in an email signature, women list their births (and losses) in a type of shorthand.

DD *3/99,* ^DS^ *6/02 28w, mmc 10/04,* one might say. This woman had a "darling daughter" in 1999, then lost a son in 2002 at twenty-eight weeks (on the baby boards, carrots around a name indicate that that baby has passed away, as the symbols look like they're pointing above), and a missed miscarriage in 2004. Or *ttc #1 since 2012. 6 mcs,* PCOS. This woman has been trying to conceive her first baby since 2012. She's had six miscarriages and suffers from polycystic ovarian syndrome, a condition common in women struggling to get pregnant.

Many of these women would love to be in my situation. Who am I to tell this tale?

But also: there is no *this* tale. The story of miscarriage is not singular. It is plural, it is various, and it is so often silent.

The *so what* of my story is that I am so afraid. I am afraid of losing this baby. I am afraid of having this baby and losing my father. I am afraid of losing them both. I am afraid of losing my mind, which some days seems like it is hanging on by the most tenuous of threads. I am afraid of postpartum psychosis and postpartum depression.

I become more and more attached to the idea of this baby.

* * *

I visited my regular primary care physician right after I got pregnant for the second time. I'm so afraid, I told him, the only thing I knew how to say.

Well, he said, that's pretty common in early pregnancy. He paused. I hear it usually goes away by the time the baby is eighteen.

It was good to laugh, to laugh together.

* * *

I tried to make my fear go away. It wouldn't. Now I try to live alongside it. It kneels when I pray. It whirls while I fret. It watches over my shoulder as I try to write again, my words coming only in short, simple sentences. It picks through the stitches while I knit a circular baby blanket, which, when finished, will look like a chunk of coral or the ocean.

I tell people about the pregnancy. I speak the news into the world like an incantation, as if the more times I say it, the more real it will become. Like in Harry Potter, how the students practice saying *wingardium leviosa, win-GAR-dium levi-O-sa,* chanting the words over and over again, until their feathers start to fly.

So: I am having a baby.

Right now this is true.

Kamali's Stillbirth

Janet Lee-Ortiz

March 30, 2017
DAY 1 OF MY STILLBIRTH STORY

I go to my regular prenatal checkup. Most of my visits have been with Kaiser's midwife, who normally just uses a Doppler. This week she is on vacation, so I'm scheduled with an OB-GYN who happens to be open for this time slot, which works with my work schedule (I hate missing work). This means I get an ultrasound today! I haven't seen baby since my anatomy scan in early January.

I'm lying down on the patient chair, and when the doctor comes in, we chitchat about how much this baby has been moving around, kicking, doing somersaults . . . those are all great signs, she says. As she gets the ultrasound going, I tell her I do not want to know the baby's sex. She sees baby's head, and she says it's in great position, head down, facing back. She measures it, measures perfectly. She scans other body parts then goes to the heart. She is having trouble finding the heart because baby's back is toward us. She thinks she finds it. I ask where it is, because I can't see it (which should have been clue number one as I know what a moving heart looks like on an ultrasound). She struggles a bit more . . . she also has trouble picking up sound. I ask her if she's kidding. She says no, let me get a

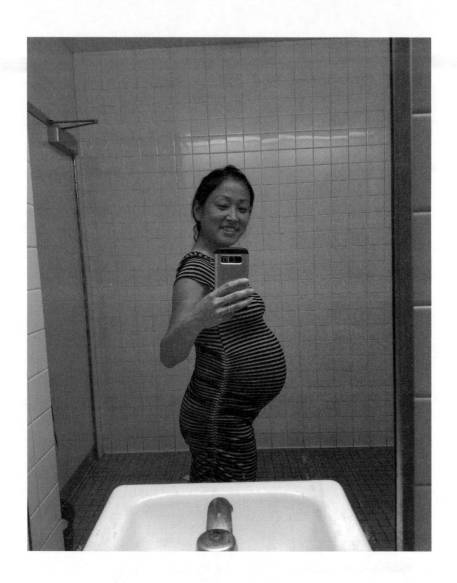

second opinion. Worry turns into panic in a split second. I'm wide-eyed and waiting for the second opinion. She asks me when was the last time baby moved. I scan my memory and think hard . . . *OH MY GOSH I don't remember it moving last night.* I feel like a horrible mother to not remember, nor did I keep kick counts. *It moved in the morning . . . but. . . . OH NO. No, no, no. . . .*

Second opinion comes in . . . she's leaning over me squinting at the screen. She grabs the device and scans me herself. She's looking and looking . . . she thinks she picks up a very faint but very slow heartbeat, but never sees movement on the heart. She looks at me straight in the eyes and says, "We need to go to labor and delivery *now.*" She grabs me by the hand, grabs my work bag, and moves at lightning speed.

I cannot soak in what is happening. It becomes a blur. I don't remember walking down, across the street, and over to the other building. During this walk I do remember asking a thousand questions back-to-back. But I also had to call my husband, call my best friend, who was supposed to be there for my birth in May, and then call work. I had to start teaching soon, but I wouldn't make it. By now I'm feeling lost and panicked. I ask the doctor, who is still leading me by the hand, if this means a C-section. She tells me if in fact there was a heartbeat, it was too slow. I asked if she could somehow jump-start the heart. I don't remember what else I asked, but I understood it either meant baby is gone or baby could come out via emergency C-section, but likelihood of survival was close to zero. I could still not comprehend how these choices could be my *only two choices.* This was all surreal, it wasn't really happening.

We make it to labor and delivery, where doctors shout at one another in a frenzy. Three doctors gather around the ultrasound machine. I'm just operating in shock mode and still not really understanding what is quite happening. They all look at the screen, another one tries . . . then suddenly, all that rushing and madness comes to a halt. All the tension in their shoulders drops simultaneously as they gaze at me, lying there with wide, questioning eyes. Finally, one of them says, "I'm so sorry."

I'm so sorry.

Then it registers. THIS IS REAL. THIS IS HAPPENING. I cover my face and lose it. Everything was going just fine. I was so close to the end, just shy of eight months. *Baby was strong and healthy. I have to start all over again? I miscarried just last year! This is a cruel, sick joke. Why did this happen?* I come in and out of waves of emotion and logical thinking. I ask them to tell me the sex of the baby since it didn't matter anymore. It's a boy. Of course, since my motherly instinct said it was a girl. I needed a name because I didn't want a blank death certificate. Taking a baby home nameless is one thing, but laying it to rest without a name is not right. I take more time to cry, because this is so so sad.

When my husband, Alex, and my first son, Essi, arrive, I'm in a private delivery room. Essi knew Mama was sad, but I could tell he was confused yet knew something was up. He stood there with eyebrows up, shrugged his shoulders, and said, *I don't know.* He did this several times. Alex and I hug, but he has to tend to Essi, and I still need more time to understand everything.

I ask the doctors what happens next. They explain how I will be induced. I want to understand each step and the names of drugs and devices used. I ask about whether I might be able to find a reason, and they tell me oftentimes there isn't a reason. When baby is birthed, sometimes there is an obvious umbilical cord issue. If not, autopsy is an option. Genetic testing looking at the DNA, rather than just the chromosomes, is another option. But often, there is no answer. I ask if I can donate its organs. Unfortunately, no. I ask if I can wait to do all this, to which they say of course, though perhaps not wait a week. All I knew was that I didn't want to stay in the hospital that day. They show me the schedule for inductions, and I decide on Sunday night, which buys me almost four full days. I choose night because the first part of induction I'm hoping I can sleep through. They tell me that in the meantime if I feel feverish or any flu-like symptoms or have signs of labor, contact them immediately. I need to go home. I need to process all this. I need to make a plan.

I get a lot done with what remains of the day. First thing is reaching out for help. I contact my doula-now-midwife and other doula friends, I connect with others who have had stillbirths, I notify friends whom I just need to ask for emotional help . . . I am able to garner a wealth of resources and get into action. Because of my emotional state, I was not able to talk to anyone. It would have been impossible to even try to complete one sentence on the phone without breaking down. Thank goodness for texting and messaging, and thank goodness for friends. I delegate and ask for help, contacting the resources provided to me. It felt like I was preparing for my own death. In a way I was, because I was going to lose a part of me forever.

March 31, 2017
DAY 2 MAKING PLANS

I wake up and hope, as with my miscarriage, that yesterday was all a horrible dream. I'm mad at myself for letting my guard down. I thought I was in the clear because I was in the third trimester. I feel like an idiot. I cry more. It doesn't feel real yet because I'm still carrying baby. I hang on to hope that there was some misdiagnosis. I think maybe by having those few additional days it will allow baby to miraculously revive itself. I believe in medical miracles. But there is definitely no movement. My womb feels heavy and silent.

Alex had fallen asleep with his head next to baby, both hands on my belly. He was certainly more spiritually connected to baby. He had a dream the night before that his own heart had stopped. Which reminds me . . . yesterday the slow, weak heartbeat that they thought they heard was most likely mine, picked up from an artery.

I don't remember what other thoughts I went through, but in the stillness of dawn and left to my own ruminations, it wasn't pretty. I text/message friends I think might be awake, because I start feeling lonely and I don't like where my head is going. I contact Midwest and East Coast

153

friends, international friends/family, people who I wouldn't be bothering so much at that hour. I know I don't have much time to be this sad because when we all wake up, I have to put on my game face for Essi's sake. I forgot where I read it, but it stuck in my mind that children shouldn't have to mourn the loss of their parents too. I didn't want him to lose the parents that he knew. Yes, I believe it is healthy for him to see my emotions, and he is very emotionally intelligent and empathetic. However, I knew it would cause confusion if I explained the loss while still visibly carrying baby. Today was not the day. So, we had to continue being the parents that he had—attentive, playful, fun, emotionally responsive, etc.

That meant SeaWorld was still on. We had promised him earlier in the week that Friday we would go to SeaWorld. During the drive I sporadically break out into tears. The news is still so fresh. I touch my belly every now and then. *How could my baby have been so alive and then suddenly gone?* At SeaWorld, we are able to operate right back into parent mode. We share laughter, have fun, enjoy one another, find joy in how alive Essi is . . . it's good for us. For dinner we grub on some good food, and I eat and drink whatever I want. At the end of the day we check into our motel and settle down for the night. Essi is being especially hilarious looking at himself and dancing very strange moves in the full-length mirror.

That's when I notice that my belly looks different. It has dropped more and become smaller. It had shrunk. It wasn't full and round. I couldn't believe the change. It made sense, as there were no fluids moving around to maintain live cells. I was in fact losing fluids in several organs. I try not to dwell on this. But at bedtime something Essi likes to do is play hide-and-seek with my protruding belly, or just hug it, or pretend parts of his face are stuck to it. When he did this tonight, it took all of me to not break apart. He won't have opportunities to do this anymore. We still had to explain to him that baby was gone.

That night I cry more. It is when I do my hardest crying. I allow myself to do this when Essi doesn't see me. In my sorrow, I'm still able to get a lot done, as I did throughout the day. My dear friends came through for

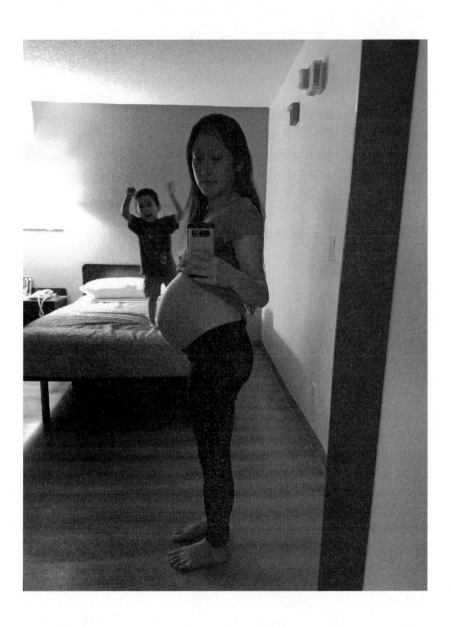

me in full force. One contacted the funeral home to arrange for cremation, another researched permits for scattering of ashes, yet another contacted a nonprofit that sends volunteer professional photographers for stillbirths. So many more were there for me emotionally. I can say I felt far from alone. I am also extremely indebted to the doulas, who were the first sources of information. They offered themselves as resources and support, and so much of me being able to just keep it together was because of them. I was able to shift my mind-set about a number of aspects in planning and preparing for this journey, namely the birth. Doulas are a special breed of people.

Some final things I did that night: Decided I needed a plan for telling people. I did not like being caught off guard yesterday at Vons when the cashier asked me, "When is your due date?" I froze, I scanned left and right searching for how to respond appropriately. In that awkwardly long amount of time that passed, she filled the space with, "Oh, you don't know." I snapped back with, "Yes, I do. It's just that . . . I . . . today I found out that . . . the baby is no longer alive." She immediately felt bad and became speechless. I scurried away and cursed to myself for being unprepared for such an interaction. I would not let it happen again. I knew I would not be able to handle an onslaught of questions and comments upon my return to work when I will clearly look different. I needed a plan for my classroom, and an age-appropriate way of telling my students. I requested the school social worker be involved to help. I asked my student teacher to please make lesson plans for the substitute.

When my head got out of work mode, I jumped right back into emotionally taking care of myself mode. I decided I wanted a piece of ash jewelry, the idea first introduced to me by a doula. At first I thought it was weird. But the more I thought about it, the more I liked the idea. I also joined a Facebook group for stillbirth support, thanks to a friend who relayed the info. I found so much support through fellow moms, many of whom had lost their angels at full term, past thirty-seven weeks. A handful had experienced multiple stillbirths. My head could not wrap around the amount of grief we all carried. Luckily, if you could call it lucky, I found the group before delivery. Most had found it afterwards. I received a plethora of helpful advice, but no one could answer my most pressing question: *How do I prepare to see my baby?* I had never held a dead body before. I had asked the doctors yesterday so I wouldn't be too shocked. They mentioned some details that I specifically asked them for, such as color and skin condition. While I tried to imagine what that might look like, I had no idea how to prepare emotionally.

No one could help me.

April 1, 2017
DAY 3 WHO WILL I BECOME?

While I didn't get much sleep, I did do a lot of research in the wee hours of the morning. My two main goals for these days were to be as prepared as possible and to enjoy the time with my family in order to experience joy in the way we knew how before being hit with life-changing grief. I needed to have some sense of control over some of this. It really did feel like I was preparing for my own death. If you've ever watched the movie *A.I. Artificial Intelligence,* what I was living felt so much like the ending of the movie when the android child is able to have just twenty-four hours more with his mom, and he was going to make every minute worth it. No, I wasn't dying. But a part of me was, and I knew I was going to come out of this experience a different person. That's what scared me.

Fear shadowed me that day. Not only was I scared of who I would become after all this, but I was also afraid of the induction and the entire labor and delivery. I knew that induced labor tends to be more intense and painful. I was afraid of the pain. I was also afraid of what the doctors had said about my placenta. They said they would gently pull on the cord to try to help remove the placenta. I did not want them to do that. I carried intense fear that something would go wrong there, that I would hemorrhage if they did that and then I would need to have a hysterectomy. Then I was mad at myself for feeling afraid of all of this, because those fears can actually get in the way of labor. I was afraid that I wouldn't be able to do it. I was scared of seeing baby and of how I would react.

It wasn't until I had a conversation with a doula that I reached an epiphany. I wasn't going in for a medical procedure. *I was preparing for birth.* This *was* a birth. I don't know why I didn't see it this way at first (in retrospect, probably because I associated birth with a live baby). Once that "aha" moment struck me, I knew what I had to do. Preparing for birth is something I knew how to do. In fact, I had already prepared for this birth . . . albeit with a *much* different outcome. All I needed to do was tweak my birth plan for . . . a stillbirth. *Right, that's all.*

Throughout the day when my friends checked in on me, I responded that I was strangely level-headed. It was kind of weird. I must have been in some sort of acceptance stage. It felt calmly reassuring, like I was doing a good job of handling all this . . . for the time being. I actually believed everyone when they told me I was strong, and that they always knew me to be strong. All the stages of grief, however, would be reset, and I'd cycle through them again once I saw baby.

Our family enjoys a nice breakfast on a perfectly beautiful day. We dine outside all together in a patio area where our dog, Nyima, was also allowed. Pancakes, French toast, eggs Benedict. Again, we share a lot of laughter and joy. I am taken aback, though, by my own profile when we pass by store windows. My belly had shrunk considerably even from just the day before. I catch myself examining my profile every chance I get. I may never see this view again.

In the afternoon we head to a dog-friendly beach in Carlsbad and hike down to the water, where we fully take in the beauty that nature offered. The only problem was that when I went to use the restroom, I had a bowel movement, at the end of which I felt strange yet familiar pressure. It was almost as if I could try to push and the baby would come out. I started to freak out. Had my water been leaking and I didn't realize it? No, my water didn't have to break for me to be in labor. I hadn't noticed any signs of labor. Did baby's head just descend farther down and was simply creating more pressure? Was my water about to break? Would I be going into labor soon? I contacted a doula and asked her for advice. My fears were eased, but I knew we had to head home. I felt I might go into labor that night.

On the drive home back to LA, I sit on a towel in case my water breaks. When we arrive home, I get straight to work on editing my birth plan and hospital packing list. I begin packing in case I need to head to the hospital this evening or in the middle of the night. Fear still lingers within me, but I push through. I'm a doer. When I set my goal on something, I try my hardest to make it happen. That level-headedness I had earlier was what carried me through the day and helped me to do what I had to do. This was the person I knew myself to be.

Would I still be her in the end?

April 2, 2017
DAY 4 INDUCTION AND LABOR

I don't remember much of the details of this day. It was just filled with lots of last-minute preparations and getting mentally ready, like getting my head into the game. Tasks were accomplished in a very matter-of-fact manner. It felt kind of like a normal day.

I know I showered. Alex played a soccer game. He also went to buy an outfit for baby so we could have the option of dressing him, though it was hard finding something small enough because I anticipated he'd be around four pounds. Both of us continued trying to find a good name. We had been looking online the past several days, but nothing was feeling right. We were the type of people who had to see the baby (or pet) before deciding on a name. The only difference in this case was that the name we eventually chose did not necessarily have to be easily pronounceable in Spanish and Korean (for our parents' sakes) as we had done with our dog and our first living child.

I also finalized details on my birth plan and printed multiple copies (for shift changes). I double-checked that I had everything on my hospital packing list. Made a run to Sprouts to put together a snack basket for the nurses. This was something I had wanted to do with my first birth, but Essi decided to come out four days sooner, so I wasn't able get it together in time.

And Essi . . . throughout all this we focused on being our usual selves for his sake. He hadn't lost his parents, and I was determined not to let that happen, though I was still afraid of what would happen after this night. When I woke up on this morning, I was reminded of how blessed we were to have him, of how joyful it was to wake up next to him each and every morning. I explained to him that tonight I would be sleeping at the hospital, and he and Daddy would sleep at home. He asked why. I explained that Mama had to go to get the baby out. *Why,* he asked. Because . . . the baby is not alive anymore. Baby died. *Why?* I don't know why, *m'ijo,* but Mama is sad. Are you sad? *No—video games!*

It was so weird to be a part of this conversation. At first I wanted to be offended. *Why are you not sad?! Why are you changing the topic when I'm trying to talk to you about something serious?* But then I realized that he doesn't see death the way we adults view death. He doesn't see it clouded with grief coupled with a deep sense of loss. He doesn't process death the same way we do. It was so interesting to witness. Later in the day I tried to bring it up again to see what he understood: Essi, where is Mama going tonight? *Hospital.* Why? *Baby dead.* Is Mama sad? *Yes.* Then he changed the topic again.

We arrive at the hospital at 8:00 p.m. It feels weird to walk in and say, "I'm here to check myself in to labor and delivery" while carrying my thirty-three-pound toddler. I'm sure the front desk folks don't see that every day. I meet my best friend, Meisha, who will be staying right beside me through this entire process. I am given the same room I was in on Thursday. Wow. Back here again. I would call this place home for two to three days, although since I'm a second-time mom, it would likely be one to two days. Part of the reason why I didn't want to stay here the day I found out was because I wasn't ready to stay for that length of time with zero preparation. The other reason was because I wanted to give my body time to naturally prepare itself for labor, namely give my placenta time to detach itself from my uterus, and hopefully allow my cervix to dilate.

I hear myself operating in a very businesslike manner. I pull out my manila folder and hand over my birth plan to the nurse. She is really sweet and gets things going in the system. I meet the doctor on duty and give her a copy of my birth plan as well. After introductions we are able to take our time to settle in. We feel quite comfortable. Alex goes to get some Thai food for dinner for all of us. It's funny, because the last meal I ate before going into active labor with Essi was also Thai. We hang out, eat, occasionally I have to answer some questions when staff come in. I have to say, the staff was incredibly respectful of our family time. But it's getting late, and Essi needs to sleep. When he and Alex leave, I immediately miss them. Despite that, I had a mission to accomplish. I had to birth this baby on my terms.

It's just me and Meisha now. When the doctor returns, we discuss our options. She explains that induction normally starts with a balloon (Foley) to open the cervix and also a dose of misoprostol to thin the cervix. Then when the cervix is "favorable," I would get hooked up to an IV and receive Pitocin to start contractions. I understand that this is standard procedure; however, I'm determined to make this birth happen with as few drugs as possible. I trust myself and my body. We discuss further, and I am somehow able to avoid getting a heparin lock (I regretted getting one with my first birth), and the doctor also agrees to start with just the balloon. So, no drugs to begin. Things are looking good because I feel like I'm getting my way already.

At 10:45 p.m., the doctor comes in to check my cervix—I'm at one centimeter—and inserts the balloon. It's not too painful, it's bearable. She explains that it can stay in for twelve hours, or if I dilate to three to four centimeters, then it will fall out on its own, which would be ideal. I tell them I want to try to sleep a bit. We agree that around 4:30 a.m. she'll return to administer the first dose of misoprostol. Sounds like a plan to me. I feel good, mostly because I don't feel like I'm being treated like a hospital patient, nor do I feel like I look like one (just a gown, which was optional, and ID bracelet). I didn't want to be hooked up to machines and fluids. A few times they mentioned the IV, but I kept pushing it, saying to do that later. I also prefer the freedom of movement during labor, so being stuck to things was not going to work for me.

Around midnight, Meisha and I get ready to sleep to prep for what's to come. I remind her to remind me to breathe through my contractions. I tell her that if she sees me losing concentration or giving up, then she needs to lock eyes with me and tell me to breathe, to do the breathing herself so I can mimic her. I remember when my doula did this with my first birth, it helped tremendously. This was a mental challenge. My head *had* to be in the game, and I had to stay focused if I was going to do this without pain meds. While I was not going to have anywhere near the outcome I had planned for, with everything in my power I was going to have the birth that I had planned for, damn it. Yes, my baby was taken away from me . . . but I was determined *not* to have the *birth* I wanted taken away from me also. I was not going to leave it to chance or fate.

I—emphasis on *I*—was going to write *that* story.

April 3, 2017
DAY 5 BIRTH AND DEATH

I fall asleep in the hospital bed just past midnight. I'm able to get about four hours of sleep. At 4:30 a.m. I wake up when the nurse comes to check on me, saying the doctor will be in shortly to administer the first dose of misoprostol. She asks how I'm feeling with the balloon, and I respond that it isn't too uncomfortable. I'm getting sporadic contractions but nothing to really indicate concern or progress.

At 5:00 a.m. the doctor comes in to administer the misoprostol. It's quick and no big deal. I try to go back to sleep because I know I have a long day ahead of me. I need the energy and all the strength I can muster, both physically and mentally. I'm not able to sleep anymore, however, so Meisha and I talk. I don't remember about what. Probably about how to help me when things pick up and about how sad all this is. Within an hour, my contractions begin to get regular. I ask Meisha to time my contractions, and she's already downloading a timer app on her phone. After timing a few, she tells me my contractions are almost one minute long at three minutes apart. Wow, that's . . . quite regular. The contractions also increase in intensity. Since it is around six o'clock and many of my friends, mostly teachers, are probably getting up by now, I text them and ask them to please send me quotes and affirmations of strength. I needed the reminders. It is getting painful already. I employ my best yoga breathing techniques and close my eyes with each contraction that comes. Each one approaches like a wave. I tell Meisha it's coming, I inhale my breath to draw in focus, then I exhale deeply to send my body the message that we are in control. In between contractions I am able to talk to Meisha and check messages on my phone. I need to draw strength from fellow women and mothers. I need to feel surrounded by my community to push through.

The contractions become more and more intense. I find myself beginning to meet some of them with fear. Those are the ones that hurt the most, and it was exactly the same case with my first birth. I knew this was a mental challenge. What made this a bigger challenge, though, was that this birth was clouded by sorrow. And I could not explain to myself or to anyone else why I needed to have a natural birth again. There was no live baby to worry about receiving residual doses of certain medications. Why did I want to do it this way? I didn't have an answer. I just knew this was what I had to do.

The hours are passing, and I'm still laboring in the bed, alternating from lying on my left side to the right side and back again. I hold on to the side rail through each contraction. Meisha is sitting next to me continuing to time each one and also applying counterpressure to my hips. I mess up on my concentration on several contractions, and I curse out loud, "Damn it, I f—ed up that one!!! Oww . . . it huuuuuurts!!!" I'm losing my mental focus. I'm feeling defeated. I can't keep going like this for hours more, probably until afternoon or evening. That is too long for me. I'm sad that I feel defeated. My mind keeps going to morphine, especially as I calculate time. The only things that seem to help are when I tell myself that it's just pressure, not pain. I also tell Meisha to tell me that, to repeat it. I ask her to please remind me to breathe. She does. She is an amazing support, and I know I could not make it through any of this without her.

At 9:00 a.m., just before the shift change, the doctor comes in to administer the second dose of misoprostol. She had explained earlier that each subsequent dose would be applied every four hours and was usually given about four times. Nevertheless, as she stands there, I explain to her that my contractions are intense and regular. In fact, they are picking up. I tell her adamantly that I do not believe I need another dose. We negotiate as my contractions continue and intermittently interrupt our conversation. In the end, we agree to hold off on the second dose until 10:45 a.m., when the balloon will be removed (twelve-hour mark). At that point we'll check my cervix to see how much progress has been made in opening and thinning it, then we'll decide if we need another dose.

The staff leaves. It's then that my body tells me to get up out of bed and move around. I had been saving my legs for when I needed them, and this was it. I get up and walk around the room aimlessly while making a sound that is a cross between a groan and a hum. I walk and sway. I am in a trancelike state. When a contraction comes, I lean over onto something and try my best to remember to breathe through it. They are painful, more than I ever remember the pain to be. I'm also not afforded the time in between to catch a breather in order to prepare for the next contraction. They have picked up. I ask out loud to no one why they are so close together, and why they hurt so much. I know what time it is, so I'm scared. If these contractions are this painful and it's only 9:30 a.m., I will certainly not make it through to the end like this. I have so much more to go. I'm not even at three centimeters, because the balloon would have fallen out of me by now. I tell Meisha I think I need to consider morphine. I need help, I can't keep going at this rate. I'm not strong enough to do this. I'm disappointed in myself and devastated that I have to deviate from my plan. I keep pushing through the contractions. I keep talking nonsense. I tell her it would be so much easier to just cut me open. I tell her I can't do this. And when I keep hearing myself say that I can't do this, I really frighten myself. Those are transition words, but I was far from transition. It was me admitting defeat.

At 10:00 a.m. I tell Meisha that I want the balloon out. I feel like it is creating additional pressure. She picks up the phone to call the nurse, and right as she does my balloon falls out. She tells the nurse, and they come in to remove the attachment from my thigh and clean up the floor. I feel slight relief of pressure but only for seconds. My mental focus is revived briefly as I tell myself I must be at least three centimeters . . . but I quickly remind myself that ten centimeters is so far to go. The contractions continue just the same as before. I want to cry. The doctor rushes in and patiently waits for me as I handle the contractions with my best breathing. I ask her to please check my cervix. I tell her I might need morphine. She waits for me to lie down on the bed, but the contractions keep attacking me with no time in between. I cry out to her that I'm so sorry, but I'm scared that if I lie down and get a contraction, I won't be able to handle the pain. She says she'll check me as quickly as possible. She is still patient as I contract while leaning over the side of the bed. I keep apologizing, and then I finally muster up the courage to throw my body onto the bed so she can check me.

"Janet, you're ten centimeters."

What?! I freeze, wide-eyed. *I'm at ten?!?!?* No wonder I was saying things that one would say during transition. I *was* in transition. This was it.

"You can push if you want. Do you want me to break your water?"

"*Yes!*—No. Wait! Someone call my husband. Someone call the photographer!"

Then I'm hit hard with the worst contraction yet. I am on my side and writhing in pain. Through my clenched jaw I groan that I can't do this, it hurts too much . . . and when I catch my breath, I realize how insane I am to even consider waiting for anyone or anything. This needed to end, and it was all right if Alex wasn't there for the moment of delivery. I plead to the doctor to please break my water. She turns around to the table of instruments to reach for the hook, but in that moment I push and break my water. I tell them I'm going to push, and they respond that I can go ahead and push. And I do. I can feel the baby's head crowning. I stop to ask if they think I will tear. Was the baby's head big? Should I push slowly to avoid tearing? I control the pushing to a medium pace and feel the baby's head come out. I push again and feel the body come out. I don't look closely at baby because the first glance I get of him I can't soak in. As baby's body rests on my lower abdomen, they clamp the umbilical cord so that I can cut it. Once cut, I ask for baby to be placed on my chest, but I turn away when I see him.

"Please cover his head," I ask through streaming tears. They get a beanie and a blanket. I look at the body and turn away again. "Please cover the parts of his skin that are . . ." I can't finish my sentence. They cover up baby more. I look once more to receive baby, and I have to turn away again. "Please rearrange his limbs so they don't look all twisted . . ." I needed him not to look like a dead body. I needed him to look like a sleeping baby. I can't stop crying. I finally hold him. He looks so frail, so peaceful, so innocent . . . I couldn't protect him.

When I snap out of it, realizing my birth isn't over, I ask if the placenta has come out. Negative. I try pushing it out. I can't. They wait. I look more at my baby, I keep hearing myself repeat, "This is all so sad. I can't believe this is my story . . ." I repeatedly tell baby that I'm so sorry. I'm reminded my job isn't done when the doctor says, "Janet, it's been twenty-five minutes. We need to get your placenta out. I'm going to pull gently to help out, though." Okay. I tell Meisha to make sure that they are indeed pulling on it gently. Yes, I say this in front of them. I push a few times. Nothing. I ask what will happen if I can't push it out. They say they will have to go in manually to remove it. My eyes widen, and I say no, I don't want that. I ask them to remind me how I need to push, where I need to focus the pushing. They said just like a bowel movement. I give one good push and birth my placenta.

And it is immediately evident: a likely link to his death. It has something to do with how the end of the umbilical cord was attached to the placenta. It was nothing that could have been detected or prevented, nothing that could have had something done about it. The doctor showed me how the cord was attached to the membrane and explained that it was slightly detached. At the time, it was reason enough to me. Something went wrong. I had suspected a cord issue, though this was something I had never heard of. It would be sent to pathology to be examined thoroughly, and a sample of my placenta would be sent to test the DNA for genetic defects, just in case. There was no rhyme or reason that this happened, so really no clear reason. (Pathology results two weeks later confirmed that there were no genetic abnormalities with either myself or the baby, and we were both perfectly healthy. But one year later I looked back at the timeline of events and realized that the only thing I had done differently was receive the Tdap vaccine, which has never been tested on pregnant women nor is there any knowledge of whether it causes fetal harm.) I was 1 in 160, which is less than 1 percent. I thank my body for knowing what to do, and I appreciate myself for listening to my body. I was able to avoid an IV, Pitocin, pain medications . . . I fulfilled my birth plan.

The staff is wonderful about granting me and my family time with baby. As time passed, his body was quickly deteriorating. When Alex arrives with Essi, he spends time with baby. He tells me that Essi understands what happened, that baby's spirit is now with the stars. Meisha, who I cannot thank enough for being by my side through all this, takes on the role of playing with Essi while Alex and I get time with the baby. We take photos, we talk, I cry, we hold him, we are present in the experience together. We take in all the little details, his perfect little hands, his big feet and long toes, his tiny eyelashes, lips that look just like Essi's . . . And Essi wants to, and gets to, briefly meet his baby brother. Hours pass before we know it. We could get all the time that we want, but baby's condition is worsening, deteriorating quickly. It is not how I want to remember him. It is time to let him go, our beautiful baby boy. We call in the staff and say we're ready.

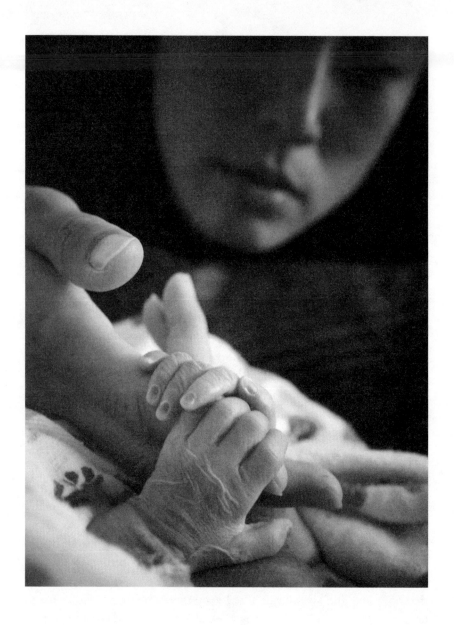

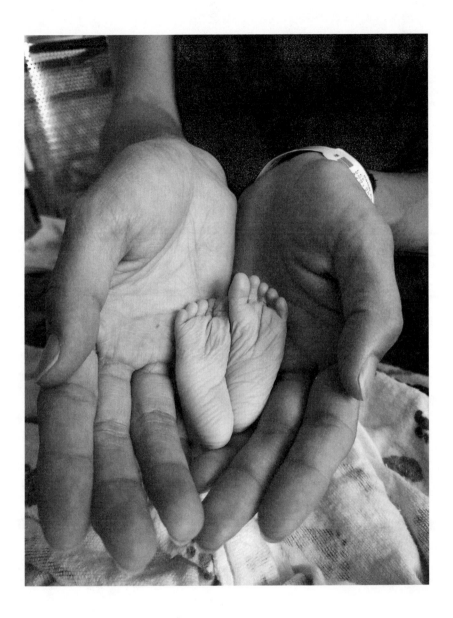

They bring in the memory box and take footprints, handprints, and hair clippings. They wrap him up and place him in a tiny burial box. To the very end, Alex and I discuss a befitting name. When they come to fill out the death certificate, we finally have a name for him.

Our baby's name is Kamali. In Arabic, Kamali means *spirit guide; protector*. His spirit will always be with us (we know, as he has shown us signs), and we will wait for him to return to us, or for us to join him.

We will always remember him. He will never be a passing memory. We will speak his name, we will share stories about him, we will celebrate his birthday and honor his life, he will forever be our son. I end my stillbirth story here, but for me there is no ending to this story. I will eternally carry with me the immeasurable grief and pain of a mother's loss.

Mama will always love you and remember you, Kamali.

Three Marias

Jen Palmares Meadows

Once, at church, a family with three daughters sat in the pew in front of ours. My father offered his hand, exchanging the kiss of peace. Three Marias, he said. That's good luck.

* * *

I pray to The Virgin now. For Grace. The room is cool, dark. An ultrasound machine makes black-and-white shadows onto a monitor. I have become wary of these examination rooms, these machines. I have known terror in wands moving over new flesh. My newborn daughter lies on her belly atop terrycloth towels, legs and arms underneath her like a frog poised to leap. Jaundice has made her unusually docile. She doesn't move when a wand strokes warm jelly along her back.

* * *

The first time, I swallowed a pill, not bothering with painkillers—staring at a wall seemed to mute my pain well enough. At first, I believed her passing would be painless, the drugs melting into my belly, sloughing away tissue like an October breeze tempting leaves from a tree. I dreamt of a girl playing. All is white space, except her laughter, which is like my sister's as a child, before I knew her. By the time I felt pain, it was too late. I curled, cried out against the expulsion. I gasped when she dropped, dared to look at that abstract bundle of tissue. I should have buried her in our backyard beneath the shade of our guava tree, should have pushed the cool dirt beneath my nails.

* * *

Our pediatrician explains it like this. The spine is made up of layers of bone, like sheets of paper one atop the other. A newborn with an indentation at the base of her spine is said to have a sacral dimple. Usually, the dimple is harmless. Other times, it indicates an abnormality called a tethered cord, wherein the base of the spine is fused together. My daughter's dimple is a shallow divot just above the rise of her bottom. It looks harmless, charming even, like a staple crimping down a too thick sheaf of papers.

* * *

The second time, I accepted anesthesia, hoping to dull the violence. They brushed tender hands over my hair and dressed me in socks, as if to offer condolences. I began to recite the states in alphabetical order. Alabama. I saw the cool wake of a clean room. Alaska. Felt the warm pressure of a hand. Arizona. I dreamt anew. Now there are two. This time, the eldest kneels to help her younger sister tie her shoelaces. I know they are girls because I weep red tears. There is laughter one moment, sorrow the next. I arranged flowers for Mary in Easter colors of purple and white. Might they know me in Heaven? I asked our priest. Go back to Galilee, he said, that place of many miracles.

* * *

Throughout the procedure, the frog sleeps, silent waves measuring her bones with moonlight. The doctor studies each image, fingers counting the pieces of her spine, dancing along the bones like piano keys. I look too, unable to discern nothing from substance, blood from bone. I wonder what he sees in these shadows sleeping in my daughter's spine. Everything looks good, he says, at last. Nothing to worry about. I hear music, caress the still sleeping frog.

* * *

When I first learned of her existence, I knelt before Mary, clutching my stomach, and said one word again and again. Please. Every day was a miracle. The holidays came, each more fearful than the last. Fear in lifting a pumpkin. Fear in placing a star. I would not leave my bed. At twelve weeks, I breathed, but did not exhale. Be careful, my mother said. You're not out of danger yet. At Easter, I saw a girl gathering eggs and wondered if I might soon hold my Maria, part her hair into black plaits.

* * *

She came to us unexpectedly. We put her in windows, wrapped her in blankets that breathed light onto yellow skin. I wept again, whispered prayers along her back. Some days, my fingers play along her spine, coaxing music from the bones there. Soon, she will twist her young body, searching for a hole in her back that might explain a strange tingling sadness, a hollow that never leaves her. And one morning, she will wake blind, eyeless. Tethered to them by sacred dimple, her hands will slide along this cord, trace it to her sisters. And when they three Marias meet at last, I will be smiling.

Susannah Wheatley Tends to the Child (Re)Named Phillis, Who Is Suffering from Asthma

Honorée Fanonne Jeffers

January 1763

When you own a child,
        can you treat her the same?
                I don't mean when you birth her,
        when you share a well of blood.
This is a complicated space.
        There is slavery here.
                There is maternity here.
        There is a high and a low
that will last centuries.
        Every speck floating in this room
                must be considered.
        I don't want to simplify
what is breathing—
        choking—
                in this room, though there are those
of you who demand that I do.
Either way I choose, I'm going
        to lose somebody.
                I want to be human,
        to assume that because Susannah

had three offspring who had died as small children—
         the details gone
                   about fevers, or coughs that clattered
         on, rashes that scattered
faces or necks or chests,
         air that did not expel,
                   never exhaled to cool tongues—
         that Susannah would be desperate
to cling to a new, little girl.
         Her need to care, her fear,
                   would rise into psalms.
         When Phillis's face
was not her mirror,
         would that have mattered?
                   When water did not drench
         Phillis's hair, but lifted it high
into kinks—
         would that have mattered?
                   Can I transcribe the desire
         of a womb to fill?
That a daughter was stolen
         from an African woman and eventually given
                   into a white woman's hands?
         And could Susannah promise the waft
of that grieving mother's spirit
         that she would keep her daughter safe
                   yet enslaved—

and this—
this—
is the craggiest
hill I've ever climbed.

The Face of Miscarriage

Soniah Kamal

I am a miscarriage veteran. The first time I miscarried I was a twenty-four-year-old newlywed, and because of a mix up in scheduling a D&C (a procedure to scrape clean the uterine lining), I'd had to keep the dead baby inside of me for two days. While I mourned the loss, I found it macabre and scary to literally be carrying death. After the D&C, I was sad but mostly relieved. Since then, I'd had several very early onset miscarriages between two live births, but nothing so traumatic.

Now at age thirty-four, I was pregnant again. After an uneventful first trimester, my husband and I joyfully announced the impending birth of our third child. Our seven-year-old son wanted a brother, and our five-year-old daughter wanted a sister. They named their new sibling Little Mo; I have no idea why. They purchased infant socks from GAP, 0–3 months, crimson with white rubber soles, and placed them on the mantle like Christmas stockings. Lil Mo's first 3-D ultrasound photo, a dimpled knot, was pinned to the fridge with a pastel magnet that spelled B-A-B-Y.

A few days later, I dropped my kids at their elementary school and headed to the Lifetime gym. My husband's job had recently moved us to Georgia, and in the absence of family or friends, bustling exercise classes were my lifeline. After the Strictly Strength class, where I did not lift more than eight pounds, I grabbed a latte and headed back home only to discover that I was bleeding. I sighed as I called the OB-GYN, who told me to come in for an ultrasound.

My husband was sad like I was, but we'd been here before. I told him to proceed to work and that I'd be fine driving myself to the OB-GYN. As I crossed red light after red light that sunny morning, I calmly readied myself for the inevitable devastation of no heartbeat. At the clinic, I was soon enough led to an exam room with the ultrasound. The OB-GYN was no nonsense as she put on her disposable gloves and had me climb onto the table and lift up my blouse. As she squirted the cold green gel onto my tummy and began to roam the ultrasound paddle over my belly, her eyes did not leave the black-and-white screen. I turned my face away and waited for the final pronouncement. And then, suddenly, the sound I least expected: the shush-shush-shush of a beating heart and the OB-GYN's proclamation: "The baby is fine!"

Still in the following weeks, heavier spells of bleeding would see me at the OB-GYN or in the ER. Each time I was assured that half of all women bleed throughout their pregnancies; it was normal, and the baby was going to make it. At home, almost every hour it seemed, I would seat myself in front of the computer and google "heavy bleeding/pregnancy/ healthy baby." Every day I would read the all the stories over and over again, drawing great solace from these first-person testimonials saying as much. There was nothing to worry about. All pregnancies were different. Some woman had bled the full nine months only to deliver perfect babies. I picked out names: Sahara for girl, and Khyber for boy.

Yet there was no way to measure how much blood was okay for each woman. A few drops, a teaspoon, a tablespoon, half a cup? How was I to know that my baby was still safe inside? And so, over the next few weeks, every time my bleeding increased more than seemed fine to me, I would panic and go to the ER. The vaginal ultrasound, a cold horrid instrument that looks like a medieval torture device, no longer hurt me; I'd grit my teeth and bear it because it was now a friend always delivering the shush-shush-shush of a heartbeat.

One Thursday evening, during a visit to the ER, a compassionate nurse, sorry I was having such a miserable pregnancy, whispered to me as they wheeled me from the ultrasound room back into the exam room that I was going to have a boy. In the exam room, the ER doctor informed my husband and me that the fetus was moving so fast, he was going to come out playing soccer.

Friday, the very next morning, the minute I woke up, I instantly knew something was very wrong. There was a lot of blood, *a lot,* more than I'd ever seen before. It tried to stay calm, remind myself that my boy was going to come out playing soccer, but something stopped me from believing it completely. Over this past month, the OB-GYN had become increasingly cold and curt, and I was usually terrified to call about anything. But this time, gathering all my courage, I dialed the clinic's number.

"Nothing is wrong," the OB-GYN snapped at me. "You're imagining things. Only last night you went to the ER, and there was a heartbeat. You're just paranoid."

"Please," I cried, "there is a lot of blood, and I won't be able to survive a minute unless I know if he's all right."

Begrudgingly, I was told to come on in then.

The bleeding plus an uncaring caregiver had unnerved me enough that I was in no state to drive myself. However, it had been my husband's turn to drop the kids at school, and he was already halfway to his office. It would have taken him longer to return in the morning traffic, and so my neighbor and friend Marilene said she would drive me.

I had thought the OB-GYN would usher me in as soon as I got there. Instead I was told to wait. I spent the next hour pacing in the reception area. Marilene kept murmuring that this was not right, and when a few women with appointments found out that I was being made to wait, they insisted that I be seen first.

In the exam room, the OB-GYN glared at me, and as I got ready for the ultrasound, she yelled at me the whole time about how much I was costing the insurance companies and that I could not just get an ultra-sound whenever I *felt* something was wrong.

Then, suddenly, she fell silent.

I knew already. My baby—Khyber—was gone. Overnight.

After the gel was cleared up, and my shirt lowered, and the OB-GYN had taken off her gloves, she led me into her office. I sat on an armchair in front of her, my eyes flicking at the wall behind her adorned with grad-uation certificates and plaques with quotes from the Bible. Her voice was back to being friendly enough, the way it had been until the pregnancy had started to go wrong. She told me that any OB-GYN could perform a D&C up to twelve weeks of pregnancy, but after twelve weeks only spe-cially qualified doctors could, and my pregnancy had been close to sixteen weeks. However, she said, the two qualified doctors in our area happened to be Jewish, and because I'd miscarried on the Jewish New Year, they wouldn't be available until Tuesday. It did not occur to me to ask her to ask them if, given the circumstances, they might make an excep-tion. It was not my job to have known to ask this.

The OB-GYN assured me repeatedly that given that just the night before there had been a heartbeat, my pregnancy hormones were simply too high for anything to happen over the weekend, and she sent me home.

The last time I'd had a dead baby inside of me, I'd felt gross and icky. This time, I treasured a final weekend to hold in my baby. Friday and Saturday were a teary blur. I was unsure of how to tell my kids that Lil Mo was gone. These past many weeks of a viable heartbeat had had me con-vinced that he was going to beat the odds. Now I didn't have the heart to take the 3-D ultrasound image off the fridge. Every half hour, I looked at the sweet knot of a face. Searched for the outline of hands, fingers, feet, toes. Finally, my husband, who believed his insistence that it was just an unviable fetus and not a baby was helpful, led to me to the living room. But there, on the mantle, were the little red socks. I kissed those 0–3 month crimson socks. I would keep kissing them every few hours, keep thinking of Hemmingway's one-line story:

For sale: baby shoes. Never worn.

Come Tuesday's D&C, I would let go; till then, I cradled my tummy.

On Sunday evening, after an early dinner where the kids ate dinosaur-shaped chicken nuggets and I picked at a few fries, I made myself a cup of chai and settled into my bed. My eyes flickered over the digital clock on my bedside table gleaming a green 5:00 p.m. as I reached for my stack of to-be-read books. I opened each book—novels, poetry, nonfiction, memoir—wishing there was some beginning that could seduce me enough so I could forget what was happening.

At exactly 7:02 p.m., I started to cramp. I sat up, experiencing the worst period pain ever, and it was only seconds later that I realized I was in the first stage of labor. The next few minutes were as if someone was turning a kaleidoscope at warp speed. While my husband called the ER—I might be in labor. Should I come in? Take a painkiller?—I was calling my next-door neighbor and friend Aruna to brief her. Could she stay with the kids until my husband and I returned from the ER? During the few minutes it took Aruna to cross her garden into mine and walk up our steps and inside my house, even as my husband ran to the garage and began backing out the car, a wave of intense pain hit me, and I rushed into the bathroom and lowered my pants and sat down.

I wish the OB-GYN had mentioned the possibility. I wish she'd warned me that if I sat on the toilet seat, catching expelled blood clots in toilet tissue, I could very well deliver my baby's face into my hands. The reason I was even sitting on the potty catching what came out of me was because my doctor mother, who lived overseas, had instructed me to catch everything I expelled in order to be able to give the D&C doctor a report.

Otherwise everything that came out of me would have simply been flushed away.

As I held his head in my palms, I could hear my husband and Aruna outside calming my scared kids, telling them that I was going to be okay.

His face was no bigger than a kitchen cabinet knob. It was opaque because cartilage is opaque. The outlines of his eyes, ears, nose, and mouth were clear. He looked like an alien out of *The X-Files* TV show. His outline resembled my older son. I can only describe the attendant wave coursing through me as aging. In those few moments, I'd accumulated decades of grief, and I felt old, forever divided between "before seeing his face" and "after seeing his face."

Should I kiss his face?

Finally, I held him to my heart and then came outside. I called the ER to update them, and then I put him in a ziplock sandwich bag so he could be sent for an autopsy. Aruna had taken my kids to their bedroom. My husband and I were silent as he drove us to the ER. The whole time I held the ziplock bag in my lap.

At the ER, I was taken to a room, and my blood pressure and temperature were taken. I was shivering and given extra blankets. My husband sat on a chair, staring at a bare wall. We were silent. According to science, it was an unviable fetus; according to my heart, it was my baby.

A chaplain held my hand and prayed with me. I told him I was Muslim, but that prayers are prayers.

I returned home that night, and the very next day onward I couldn't stop sharing the story of my miscarriage. I told neighbors I'd exchanged mere nods with. I would tell the cashier at the grocery store. While my kids were at school, I would telephone my family, who all lived overseas. I called my close friends, all of whom lived in other states. It was as if I was confessing and my confession had opened gates to a taboo subject. Family, friends, neighbors, strangers—everyone came out. Either they shared their story of their own miscarriage or else someone else's. It turned out that even my mother had miscarried before me.

Everyone kindly reminded me, over and over again, that I already *had* two kids. I could have another one. As if babies are replaceable. That I'd been barely sixteen weeks. Too many said, "It wasn't a stillbirth. You weren't full term. Stop being so sad!" No one, not even my husband, could quite understand why I was so gutted. Fetus, he kept telling me, unviable fetus.

Their words left me upset, alone, and angry at having conditions put on grief and attachment.

My kids knew something was wrong. Each time I saw them, my eyes would well up. Each time I saw them I thought: If I can't keep a baby safe inside of me, how am I going to protect these two who are out and about in the world?

One afternoon, soon after the miscarriage, as my kids cleaned out their Spiderman and Dora the Explorer backpacks, I blurted out,

"Lil Mo is gone."

"Gone?" said my son.

"He died."

My son's best friend's father had passed away, and so my son had an inkling of life after death: Dylan's father was in heaven, and heaven was a good place.

"So Lil Mo's in heaven?" His eyes filled up. "Like Dylan's father?"

"Yes," I said, and as I looked into his eyes, I knew that whether heaven existed or not, it belonged more to him than me in that moment, to little children confronted with mortality.

Over the next month, we began to recover, if recover is the correct sum of time plus distance that allows for healing. My husband stopped saying "fetus" even if he couldn't say "baby." We discussed how before pregnancy tests, women had to miss up to three to four periods before they could confirm a positive result and that if they miscarried, they might just mistake it for erratic periods, but now, thanks to the early testing, women could get attached at conception even.

One evening, without even realizing I was going to do so, I took Lil Mo's ultrasound picture off the fridge. My son put it in his album that held pictures of his beloved dead guinea pigs. I took Khyber's crimson socks off the mantle and tucked them at the back of a drawer that held my own socks. What was done was done. Despite being told that he would come out playing soccer, my baby was gone, and I had to survive in a world where for the one month I'd bled, I'd yet believed that he would make it, that he was a survivor.

Around a month after the miscarriage, I received a call from Northside Hospital: What did I want to do with the remains?

I had not realized there would be "remains."

The very word *remains* brought back every little bit of grief that I thought I'd dealt with.

I replaced the cordless in its cradle with shaking hands.

He was dead, and there were remains.

Muslims bury their dead. My husband called the local mosque. He was informed that there could be no burial. In Islam it is believed a soul enters the body at around 120 days (sixteen weeks), and since my miscarriage took place right around that time, there was no proof that a soul had indeed entered; what had been inside me could only safely be considered a soulless fetus.

Fresh raw grief sliced me open. My husband was quiet. He said we could do whatever I chose to do with the "remains." I took a cordless phone into the guest bathroom where I'd delivered Khyber's face into my hands, and I telephoned my support at Northside Hospital's perinatal loss clinic. She was a kind, gentle nurse with whom I'd so far exchanged emails about how the OB-GYN had made a terrible situation so much worse with her callousness. In the nurse's latest email to me, she'd written that she'd seen my baby's remains and that he'd been beautiful. There was no thank-you that could have ever conveyed my gratitude for her saying that.

"Please," I said to her now, "please don't throw him in the trash."

"Of course not," she said. And then, very tenderly, "The hospital takes the remains of such babies for a collective cremation. Would you consider that?"

As soon as she said "collective" and "cremation," I recalled a trip to the Holocaust Memorial Museum in D.C. I recalled a blown-up photo of a funeral pyre with limbs sticking out. I did not want my baby to be one of many. And yet the human mind is such that, within hours, I found comfort in the very idea of a collective. That way, I comforted myself, Khyber would at least never be alone.

Friday, October 12, 2007, 6:28 p.m.: <*pnl@atlanta.com*> wrote:
Directions to Stone Mountain Cemetery: The cemetery is located in old town Stone Mountain at the corner of Ponce de Leon Avenue and James B. Rivers Drive. As you drive into the cemetery, take the road on your right. You will pass some Confederate soldier markers. Make the 2nd right, which will dead end into another small road. The plot where the babies are buried is the site on the right across the road in front of you. It has a very large oak tree shading it on the right side.

A few weeks later, on a cold but sunny October day, my husband printed out the directions the nurse had emailed, and he, I, and our kids set out for the cemetery in Stone Mountain. In the car, the kids chattered about Halloween and how this year they were going to use pillowcases to trick or treat. When we neared the cemetery, they quieted, and there was absolute silence as we drove through lanes between U-shaped headstones, many adorned with wreaths.

My husband took a second right and then another right into a small lane. We saw the plot immediately. It was the size of a small rectangular swimming pool enclosed within gray brick ankle-height boundaries. We parked beside the plot. The collected ashes of all miscarried babies were buried in the plot, which was shaded at one side by a lone oak tree. There were a few bouquets along the sides of the plot.

You will also find a small marble bench with a carved dove on it there. This was donated and is the only memorial that is allowed to mark the presence of the babies who have died. Please feel free to rest on the bench while visiting the gravesite. If you have brought flowers, please use the vase at the side of the bench as a place to put them.

My son had brought as an offering a miniature teddy bear I'd given him for Valentine's Day, and my daughter, a rose from our garden. They placed them by the oak tree, and then we walked to the bench, which was directly opposite the oak tree. The bench was hewn of simple rough stone, a slab for a seat and two slabs for feet. The slab feet were half taken over by overgrown grass. A dove carrying an olive branch was carved into the center of the front side of the seat slab. I settled in the middle of the bench, my knees covering the dove, my kids sitting on either side of me, my husband perched behind us. We sat for a while. I recited a prayer for my baby. I recited a prayer for all the babies.

A Dream Deferred

Marcie Rendon

What happens to a dream deferred?
    Does it dry up
    like a raisin in the sun?
    Or fester like a sore—
    And then run?
    Does it stink like rotten meat?
    Or crust and sugar over—
    like a syrupy sweet?

Maybe it just sags
like a heavy load.

Or does it explode?

    —Langston Hughes, "Harlem"

Life ignites into being. A flash signaling existence exactly at the moment of conception. Denied by those less knowing. But I knew. Each time. I knew. That moment. That flash. When I was no longer one being but two.

1972. Twenty-two, madly in love and desperate for family, I sat in my car and watched a train pass by. My stomach churned. It was the only moment of morning sickness I ever remember experiencing. It was the time before warning about alcohol consumption. No one talked about the effects of smoking on the infant growing internally. I knew nothing other than my own desperate longing and love.

Five months along I was sitting in a movie theater in Denver. Summer break from college. Unmarried, with a boyfriend whose boarding school–raised Catholic mother was not only unhappy with my existence in her favored son's life but who also had some very heavy judgments about an illegitimate child on the way.

Midway through the movie I felt a hot rush of thick liquid fill my jeans. I had no idea what was happening, and it didn't occur to me to engage the three other young adults who were sitting in the theater with me that evening. I got up and walked the few short blocks to my boyfriend's parents' house and upstairs to the bathroom. It was in the bathroom light that it was obvious the liquid on my jeans was blood. Looking back, I can only imagine I was in emotional shock. I didn't feel sick. I didn't feel faint. Rather a numbness overtook me. I changed out of my jeans and went downstairs and told my boyfriend's mother and his aunt that I had just lost my baby.

There was no change of expression on either of their faces. I remember them looking at each other as I stood there, blood filling the sanitary pad I had put on. The aunt got up and said, "I'll give you a ride to the emergency room." Which she did. She dropped me off, and I walked in alone.

I don't remember the lonely wait. Nor the D&C the doctor performed to remove all "tissue." I do remember the early morning darkness I walked home in. Nine blocks of early morning darkness after the loss of a child and a D&C. Again, numb with emotional shock. At the house I crawled into bed and stayed there for two or three days. No one, other than my boyfriend, mentioned the baby I mourned for.

Summer passed. I resumed drinking and partying as if all were normal. My boyfriend and I still madly in love. We finished each other's sentences. Laughed together at jokes only we understood. His arm was always around my shoulders, mine around his waist. It drove his father crazy. And his Catholic-raised mother even crazier.

College started in September, and I began classes. One day that fall I was sitting with a group of friends in the student union. My boyfriend was making jokes. Everyone was laughing, talking. Having a good time. Without warning, with no sense of impending doom, for me the room went dark. Where before the room had been filled with sunshine pouring in the windows, the entire room now turned gray. I looked at everyone sitting at the table. No one else seemed to notice. But for me, the room remained devoid of color. Devoid of the sunshine I knew was shining outside the windows.

I finally gathered the courage to ask my friend sitting next to me, "Did the lights go out in here? Is it dark in here?"

She looked at me kinda funny and said, "No," and rejoined the laughing conversation. I got up and left the group, waving a hand at my boyfriend that meant go ahead and stay. Even walking home to our apartment, I logically knew the sun was shining, but the entire world was gray.

At twenty-two, I had never been to therapy. I had never taken a psychology class. I had no framework for what was occurring, but I knew things were seriously bending out of reality's shape.

Within that week I withdrew from classes and moved to a friend's cabin on the reservation, where I remained for the rest of the semester. Deep in grief, I cried and wrote and sat for hours by the edge of the lake. Sometimes I watched the sun come up. Sometimes I watched the sun go down. Other times it was the moon that kept me company. My boyfriend would come by periodically to see if I was ready to return. We were still madly in love. On his visits he would lie in bed with me and hold me, just hold me. Other times we would get into the boat that was tied at the dock, and he would row us out into the middle of the lake, where we would lie in the bottom of the boat and float the afternoon away until the evening mosquitoes arrived and chased us back to shore. Sunday night he would ask if I wanted to come home with him, and I would say no.

I don't remember how long I stayed there, but I do remember I returned to school before the snow fell. We got married before he graduated. I graduated a year later. Together we had two beautiful daughters. With the pregnancies I ceased drinking. His consumption increased. He continued to work and party and I parented. The madly in love changed to "Oh my god, how do we survive the addictions?" We didn't. We got divorced. Seven years later I made the bold decision to have another child on my own. Another beautiful girl.

After single parenting for a few too many years, I remarried with the idea, the goal, of having at least two more children, but this time with a partner.

I remember the first conception with husband number two. We had just made love, and I felt the familiar "ping" of existence pop into being. I knew. We were both very happy, as our goal for parenting and married life was moving ahead on schedule.

Unfortunately, that was not the plan of the universe. It was evening. He was teaching at a campus an hour away. My three daughters and I were home with another friend of the family. I felt a pain in my lower right side. As the evening wore on, the pain became intense. The pain became excruciating. I couldn't bear anyone touching me. I felt like an animal caught in a trap, ready to attack even the rescuer who tries to free it. Finally, my friend convinced me I needed to go to the hospital. She would drive.

The three girls went down and got the car doors open. They all three squished in the front seat. Still unable to be touched, to have anyone within three feet of me—that is how far the pain radiated out of me—I crawled down the stairs. We lived in an upstairs duplex. I crawled on the sidewalk to the car. I remember seeing an old boyfriend walking down the sidewalk. He ignored me. In my pained state I had to stop and hold myself in a ball on the sidewalk so as not to laugh as I imagined him going to an AA meeting and reporting seeing me crawling drunkenly down the sidewalk.

At the hospital I was rushed into emergency surgery for an ectopic pregnancy.

As I recovered in the hospital, my doctor assured me the tube had not ruptured. That I would still be able to get pregnant. The tubes were open and functioning. She couldn't give me a reason as to why this baby had decided to stop midway home.

Two more ectopic pregnancies. Two more emergency surgeries.

The last ectopic pregnancy sent me into physical shock. My blood pressure dropped. I was on the verge of dying at home before the ambulance arrived and wrapped me like a tin-foiled hotdog at the state fair. I learned later it was a blanket to help my body handle the shock it was going through.

As I was going in to surgery for the third time, I told my doctor to have a spiritual advisor waiting for me after I woke as I didn't know how I would cope with losing this third baby.

She did have someone waiting to talk with me. He just wanted to pray over me. My doctor had much better guidance than he. As I lay in the hospital bed recovering, once again, living in a world of gray, my doctor told me to stop trying to get pregnant. She told me all tests still showed two viable, functioning fallopian tubes, and she could give me no medical reason as to why my babies were getting stuck on their way to this existence. She told me that maybe the Creator had a higher purpose for me at this time in my life than to give physical birth. She suggested in vitro fertilization as one option to have more children, and she also suggested adoption. I was open to either. My husband wasn't. We divorced shortly after.

Each ectopic pregnancy had thrown me into deep grief, but prior to the last one there had always been hope. As I left the hospital the third time, I was ready for the grief. I told myself I would grieve as long as I needed to reach full acceptance that my days as a creator of children were over. That my dream of an even larger family to love was dashed, finished. That I would grieve the loss of babies, the loss of life, the loss of hope, the loss of dreams, the loss of family. I would grieve until I knew what other plan the Creator had for me. I would grieve fully, completely so that as a woman I could continue to create.

I don't know where else to put this in the story. With each surgery for the babies, my doctor saved the fetus for me to bring home. As a family we held a burial for each tiny being at a place by moving water that felt like home to me. A place that I could visit if pulled to do so.

But rather than stay at the resting place I found for them, the spirits of those little ones followed my family for years. They would hang around the doorway of my house, and whether you believe it or not, at least three people became pregnant after visiting our family overnight.

And myself? I became a full-time writer. Pouring my creative energy into stories, poems, plays, and novels.

Pity

Seema Reza

The first time I decided to have a second child, I was following convention. Our older son would be five by the time the new baby was born. It
was time. My husband, Karim, was ready, and so I agreed. I was ready to
buy a new house, decorate a new room—maybe in pink. I was ready to be
pregnant and eat more cake. But I was reluctant to introduce myself as the
mother of two.

One child is okay. One child will fold himself into the back seat of a
two-door coupe. But *two* children? Two children require more car, less living room, a big backyard. Two children suggest you're in it for good. It is
harder to find babysitting, harder to have sex, harder to be *you* with two
children. So I wasn't 100 percent thrilled. Though I knew it was the right
thing for my life. A decision Karim and I would not regret.

I was pregnant before we really tried. Before I had even laid all these
thoughts out.

I was so *charmed* that he wanted another baby. And flattered, validated
as a mother. He wanted another baby with *me*. So I was pregnant. And determined to take pregnancy in stride. I was twenty-four. Healthy. *Pregnancy
is not a medical condition.*

We went on hikes and on long bike rides. I drank tea (caffeinated), gave
piggyback rides, went to concerts and the pumpkin patch. I didn't throw

up. I didn't feel too tired. I hardly felt pregnant at all. I went to prenatal appointments, prepared four-year-old Sam for the new baby. *A baby is great,* I told him. *A baby will make you laugh and be your friend. A baby will be the best thing that ever happens to you.*

He was sometimes skeptical but mostly uninterested. I took him to hear the heartbeat for the first time. He held my hand and cringed when my blood was drawn and smiled shyly at the attention from the doctor and nurses.

Sam was at school when the first call came. Karim was at the kitchen table, repairing his glasses with a tiny screwdriver. I was flipping through a catalog.

The nurse said my AFP test numbers came out too high for my eighteen weeks. There was too much alpha-fetoprotein from the baby's liver in my blood. Something about a possible neurological defect.

Or maybe twins, I countered. *I read the pamphlet.*

She scheduled me for an ultrasound with a specialist forty-five minutes away. I researched AFP. Called my sister. Cried. Hyperventilated. Felt melodramatic for overreacting.

I didn't tell my parents—they had a vacation planned at the time of the test, and I hated to worry them for what would surely turn out to be nothing. Karim was starting his end-of-year use-or-lose-leave-time vacation the Friday of the appointment. It made sense to start the vacation by getting this cleared up. Everyone assured me everything would be okay. I agreed.

The doctor's waiting room was a bare rectangle. Walls lined with chairs upholstered in mauve. I was tempted to leap from chair to chair while I waited.

I was having twins! Or maybe my due date was earlier than the thus far predicted May. I filled out the form. A genetic *Cosmo* quiz.

Are you Jewish, Hispanic, over thirty-five? Are you and your spouse related? Do you have any history of genetic problems in your family?

We aced the test. All noes. Congratulations, you're having a healthy baby.

The waiting room began to fill. There was a Hispanic couple with a three- or four-year-old daughter. There was an older couple. Waaaay older. I felt sorry for them. I nudged Karim and whispered, *There must be something wrong with their babies. They must have failed the questionnaire.* He nodded in agreement.

We went in and met the doctor. Bald and unfriendly and delicate, he performed the ultrasound silently in the cramped, dark room. He didn't make small talk, didn't point out the baby's body parts. He kept the screen to himself. We thought he might have social problems.

He left the room (my belly sticky and exposed) and came back with a nurse in pink scrubs. She ran the machine. She left the room.

He came back. *The prognosis is not good.*

I was still smiling to encourage the doctor's social skills.

There's very little amniotic fluid. Terminate. Soon. You're young. Have another baby later. Are you leaking fluid?

I wasn't.

Your outcome won't be good, You have to decide soon. Before it's too late to be legal.

At some point, I dropped my smile, refused to accept it. Demanded a rematch with another ultrasound machine. They worked us into the schedule for Monday. We walked out through the waiting room, tears streaming. And the couples waiting must have felt so sorry for us.

The hours after you get bad news are like airplane turbulence. The weightless rise on the first impulse to convince yourself that you misheard, that the information was faulty. The grasping and scrambling on pure air. And then the down side, the drag: when you're yanked down from your gut and you just want to fold.

I rested my head against the cold window of the car, letting it bounce against the vibrating, buzzing glass. Karim drove fast, expertly, left-handed. His right hand was in my lap, enclosing my left hand, almost touching my rounding belly. Several times words formed in my mouth, and when I released them, they bounced between us, as hollow as tennis balls.

My oldest sister, Mona, picked Sam up from school that first day. She had made beef Stroganoff (my craving) and bought sparkling cider to celebrate the inevitable all clear. When she answered the phone, I echoed the doctor: "The prognosis isn't good."

When I hung up, she called our parents back from vacation, called our aunt and uncle in Baltimore, put away the sparkling cider.

It was dark in her living room. Mona had recently moved, and the room was empty aside from an ornate bench and an opulent rug. I sat on the edge of the bench and dialed my aunt the pediatrician.

When she answered, I stood and traced the edge of the rug with clockwise steps. I told her what the doctor had told me and then answered all her questions.

The fluid is low. Five cc's. Eighteen weeks. High AFP. Dr. Khrusey. I'll have another sono on Monday.

She didn't offer her classic you-are-overreacting irritation, didn't explain how it was really not such a big deal. Just told me to prepare for a difficult journey.

I canceled the follow-up appointment scheduled for Monday. I went to better appointments arranged by family and friends with prominent doctors; doctors with websites and publications.

We saw the beautiful doctor whose waiting room was packed full of pregnant women grumbling with discontent at Food Network on the television. When she performed the ultrasound, she turned a little screen toward me so that I could see as well. With the fluid so low, there was only gray, with the steady pulsing of a small heart in its midst. Then she held my hand and cried; she had lost a baby of her own just months before. Her nurse cried too. Karim kept his eyes wide and dry and asked questions.

We had another appointment after that, with Johns Hopkins doctors— *the best of the best.* The Hopkins doctors were narrow and intellectual and striking. They didn't wear makeup, didn't seem to brush their hair. They wore sweaters and socks of thick, practical wool with their scrubs. They gave us a jewel of hope and put me on light bed rest for a month. Karim gave a homeless man a twenty on the way home, succumbing to superstition after years of cocky agnosticism.

On bed rest, I watched every movie anyone recommended: *The Royal Tenenbaums, The Life Aquatic.* I fell asleep during *Star Wars* three times, until Karim gave up. I wet the bed a few times, woke hopeful, and went to the doctor thinking the fluid leak mystery had been solved, that we might finally know where it was going.

While I was inert, a tsunami in South Asia caused hundreds of thousands of deaths and left families devastated. I avoided the news, but Mona was obsessed, so the stories reached my ears. Against my will, it put my woes in perspective, all these people drowning on land. But inside my body my child was withering, the amniotic sac clinging to its limbs like a plastic bag.

According to the Internet, some babies with oligohydramnios in early pregnancy do make it. The baby was active, that was unusual, surely a good sign. I was drinking bottles upon bottles of water. I lay on my left side, removed caffeine from my diet completely. Pomegranate juice was supposed to be good, and I drank a tart cupful every afternoon. I tried anything that was recommended. Except for God. If he existed, he was clearly overwhelmed.

After my month was up, I went back to Johns Hopkins. Nothing had changed; my baby was still alive, the fluid was nearly nonexistent. A decision might have to be made after all. During the ultrasound, the doctor found that the baby had a cleft lip and palate. That was the first solid thing wrong with the baby.

Before that it was the fluid, only the fluid, and so many guesses on how the low fluid might affect the baby. The bladder appeared to be filling and emptying, and "practice breathing" was evident, and we saw sucking motions, and the baby was moving, moving. So it seemed like maybe the fluid was *their* problem, not ours. But the cleft lip and palate made three things wrong, and miracles more elusive.

I underwent genetic testing. The testing rooms at Hopkins are cavernous, sterile cubes of gray. They rubbed iodine on my belly and in dim light punctured my abdomen with a long needle and, guided by ultrasound, led it into the placenta and pumped in and out. Hard. I welcomed the pain. Everyone was so nice, so compassionate. But I remembered the things I'd done wrong:

I hadn't been off the pill for long before I got pregnant (two weeks).

I had a couple of drinks (five weeks).

I had to stop to breathe during a tough bike ride (ten weeks).

I lost control of a fight with Karim (fifteen weeks).

I went to a concert in a smoky bar (seventeen weeks).

I was bad about prenatal vitamins (most weeks).

The apricot placental tissue was sucked into the syringe, and my uterus cramped. As the iodine was wiped from my belly and the lights were turned up, the doctor said:

"Take it easy today and back to normal activity tomorrow."

"No bed rest?"

"It didn't seem to help, so no."

Even the best of the best were giving up.

After putting Sam to bed, I brought the CD player from my bedside table into the bathroom and plugged it in next to the sink. I pressed play, turned the volume up, filled the tub halfway with warm water, and climbed in. I held my breath and lay down face first, checking that my ears were fully submerged, balancing my weight on my folded elbows to keep the pressure on my belly minimal. The edge of the drain plug pressed into the top of my head. I could hear long notes of music playing through the water and the garbled lyrics. When I pushed myself up on to my arms, the air felt sharp against my face and neck, the music seemed too loud. So I took another breath and lay back down.

Seema. SEEMA.

I turned on to my side to see Karim kneeling at the side of the tub on one knee. I pushed the wet hair from my face and smiled at him.

He put his face in his hands and shook his head, then looked up. I could see white all the way around his brown irises. "Why?"

"Oh. Sorry." I realized what he thought he had walked in on. "I wanted to hear what the baby hears. There's not really this much fluid in there, but there's fluid in the rest of my tissue. I think the baby can hear me singing. I think it hears you too." I pulled the knob, and hot water rushed into the tub. When the water level rose to the overflow drain, I raised my foot and pushed it off. "I'm not suicidal. Are you?"

He furrowed his brows. "No. Why would I be?"

"Why would I?"

Karim sat on the lid of the toilet. He gave me a half smile through the rising steam, and I missed him. I missed the crinkles at the corners of his eyes when he laughed, and I missed hearing what he really thought. I missed his old confidence, his I-can-solve-anything attitude. I missed making plans. We scheduled only as far as dinner tonight, what movie we should watch next. Each unwilling to bring up the topic our lives spun around lest the other be reminded of it in a rare moment of peace.

I unplugged the drain. Karim passed me a towel and steadied me as I stepped over the side of the tub. I stood in front of him, and he rested his head against my damp body.

I protected my baby—there wasn't any fluid there to cushion my movement. I walked slowly to avoid jostling. Karim suggested tying pillows around my middle. I laughed. He wasn't joking.

My cousin was getting married, so rather than risk slipping in heels, I ventured out to buy flat dress shoes, a first in my adult life.

In the mall I felt absurd, conspicuous. Like a bear posing as a person. I felt certain that someone would stop me and tell me that I should be home crying. Karim walked beside me, his hand at my elbow. Within fifteen minutes I bought my shoes and left the mall. Another first.

My mouth always tasted unwashed, my hair lay flattened on one side. Deep circles had carved space under my eyes, and my cheeks were swollen from so much unearned sleep. A fog clung to me. I donned silk, lipstick, jewelry. The reflection of the sequins on my clothes made me wince.

The wedding was held in a plush ballroom adorned with chandeliers, yards of tulle and vases of flowers set on pedestals. At any point, the doctors told me, I was likely to become a tomb. I hadn't felt the baby move for a day and a half by the evening of the wedding. I smiled in pictures, ate what was served, congratulated the happy couple—all the while moving through syrup. I avoided adult conversation, and when it found me, my responses were mumbled and peculiar. Karim spent the evening taking photographs of our nieces, nephews, and son. Each time our eyes caught, he tilted his head to the side, and I shook my head.

And when finally, on the car ride home we played music loud and I felt distinct kneading against the inside wall of my abdomen, I was not entirely relieved.

We met with a genetic counselor. Her office had two tweed chairs for us to sit in. I noted the placement of the tissues. There were tissues everywhere these days. Everyone expected me to cry.

While she asked us about our families' medical history, Karim sat at the edge of his seat, jiggling his far leg. I couldn't feel it, but it annoyed me. We offered my grandmother's cancer, my father's thyroid, Karim's grandfather's heart attack and early demise. Karim offered an autistic cousin, which seemed to pique her interest.

She showed us a chart of neatly arranged tooth-shaped chromosomes and told us about trisomy 23 and spina bifida. She told us adoption was an option.

At home it was back to the Internet. We googled cleft lip. It's not a big deal, it can be corrected. There'll be a little scar above the lip, but so? Cleft palate gets trickier.

I drew my tongue across the roof of my mouth. The joint jutting out would be missing in the baby's mouth. So the baby wouldn't be able to drink milk without a feeding tube. Breastfeeding—my magic trick—would not happen. A chunk of my resolve broke off and floated away. We began to divide.

When you die, Karim would tell me, *I will have you cryogenically frozen.*

When you die, I invariably responded, *I will have you buried.*

In eighth grade, I told the class that I was pro-choice for everyone, but pro-life for me. In tenth grade, a friend of mine was on her second abortion. I hit the prayer mat, reaching out to a God I had been on the outs with for years. In eleventh grade, I took a pregnancy test in the girls' bathroom at school and was relieved to have no decision to make. The following year my grandmother, watching my trash can like a hawk, noticed that I hadn't had my period in two months. I used tampons, which she did not recognize. She offered to take me for a quiet abortion. In college I discovered science. I pored over the laws of chemistry. For once, it made irrefutable sense. I took astronomy, calculus, physics—with each course, guilt over my doubts lifted until I was finally free of God. And then this.

Everyone told me to pray. There is a special prayer, the *Istikara,* Muslims use to help make decisions. A specific Quranic verse is recited just before bed, and the correct path is revealed in dreams. In short, have a nightmare, and forget it. Have a happy dream, and go for it. I wanted to believe that if God wanted my baby, He would take him. That I just had to wait, and it would all unfold. If I did lose the baby, we would eventually be reunited, and I would see it take its first steps in heaven. But I had seen a fair bit of His handiwork and had no confidence in His thought processes. So the decision would have to be mine.

Karim and I discussed it gently, one of us retreating when the other became agitated. He brought me articles from the Internet—babies who had made it. I carefully highlighted the differences between their cases and ours. I was *not* leaking fluid, our baby was younger, my fluid was lower. I had pored over these same articles, had asked the doctors many of these questions. I pointed out that while *the doctors said the baby was going to die horribly and then he did* was not a particularly compelling or interesting story, it was probably the more common one.

The uncomfortable truth was that it was ultimately my decision. While Karim was pleading with me to keep his baby alive, I thought of the baby, gasping for air like a fish out of water. I thought of Sam, burdened for life with a younger sibling who wouldn't be a companion. I thought of Karim, already stretched, trying to juggle the added expense and stress of a very sick child. I thought of myself, consumed forever with childcare and destined for a ponytail and untamed eyebrows.

One day, between movies, my cousin and I happened upon an episode of *Oprah*. Her guest that day was Mattie Stepanek's mother. Mattie was born with dysautonomic mitochondrial myopathy and passed away just shy of his fourteenth birthday. His mother spoke of his last moments: the intensity of his pain, the deterioration of his body as his muscles distorted and twisted him from within, causing him to lose his hair and fingernails while she begged him to stay alive for her. She spoke of his amazing accomplishments, his poetry and speaking engagements, and the lives he touched. She didn't regret a moment of it. All I could think of was Mattie's fingernails falling off.

When I finally made the decision, it seemed so sudden—they told me it was a boy, they told me he was starting to get clubbed feet, they told me there was no hope. Hope was starting to feel like a selfish luxury, and so I succumbed. I wanted this over. I wanted to be with Sam, to make pancakes with him and enjoy his four-year-old wisdom instead of shuffling him from family member to family member. I wanted it to end.

I had seen all the pieces before—the low-fluid ultrasound, the sharp, stark line of the needle as it enters the image on the screen. Though they turned the screen away from me, I could see it all. Karim watched the screen. He held my hand, but my guilt and his uncertainty made the motion feel automatic.

I wanted to shut my eyes, but I forced myself to look at Karim's face. His jaw was clenched, his eyes wet. The needle went in, full of adrenaline. I imagined it piercing through the soft, unformed fetal breastbone, entering the heart that I had seen pulsing rapidly at my first prenatal appointment, the heart that I had lain in examining rooms listening to.

Oh. The doctors (residents really—doctors are reserved for life *saving*) whispered among themselves briefly. They prepared a second needle.

It didn't work? I considered reconsidering. Was this a sign? Should I just get up and run, leave my shoes, my purse, my pants? In went the needle again, and this time it worked. Karim let go of my hand. I shut my eyes, and they cleaned me off, turned on the light and began to tidy up. I put on my maternity jeans.

They led me down a long hallway with no doors. Behind me were the series of passageways that led to the ultrasounds, the examining rooms, the genetic counselors' offices. Before me, the nurses' station in the blue-tiled labor and delivery ward shone.

Pulling a twenty-three-week-old fetus from the womb is not simple. First, a steady drip of Pitocin is fed into the bloodstream to induce contractions. One thousand milligrams of Tylenol are also administered to fight the inevitable fever that arises when the body resists relinquishing the baby. Next, to begin the dilation of an unwilling cervix, toothpicks of seaweed are forced into the tight tissue every hour or so.

I watched CNN during my first seaweed treatment. With studied focus, I read the ticker tape to the doctor and nurse, and we discussed current events like friends.

Karim stood by the bed, folding and unfolding his arms and staring at the television. When the doctor and nurse left the room, he sat next to me on the bed, and I pressed my face into his neck. His warm skin smelled of home.

I felt the baby twitch and brought my hand to my stomach. *Rigor mortis?*

After a few hours, the Pitocin began to kick in. Another drip was attached, this time with morphine. The nurse handed me a button that would release the painkiller into my blood. My fever spiked, and I began to vomit.

Mona, who had brought our mother along after arranging childcare for Sam and her own daughters, tied my hair back with a child's turquoise flowered tie pulled from the depths of her purse. My mother looked frightened and hollow. Karim held the kidney-shaped bedpan under my mouth until I lay back.

I opened my eyes, needing to vomit again. *Karim, the thing. I need the thing.*

The room was amber and blurred. I heard only shuffling and murmuring. They couldn't understand me, and I growled louder, frustrated, my mouth felt full of rocks, my jaw twitched. The effort to speak exhausted me, taxed my diaphragm. I had a faint impression of the bedpan being passed from hand to hand until Mona or Karim or my mother was holding it in front of me. I retched and lay back.

Time passed. One nurse left, another began her shift. The contractions started to come. I still had not used the morphine. I was in control of that, swallowing the pain.

A few times I opened my eyes, and the room was quiet. Two people had left the room, and the third was snoring softly on the chair in the corner. I had nothing left to offer the bedpan, so I sat in the dark with my hands folded under my belly until sleep took me again.

As night began to give over to morning, the contractions came closer together. Karim had just fallen asleep, and I hated waking him. He stood and rubbed his eyes with his fingertips, disoriented. The shake of his head, the crush as he brought himself to the present made me fully conscious for the first time in eighteen hours.

This is usually the exciting part. He came and stood to the right of the bed, pressed the back of his hand against my cheek.

My sister and my mother stood behind him, near my head, and I heard my sister whisper to my mother: *You can stay, but do not gasp.*

I pressed the button twice, ready for the morphine.

The gentle doctor whom I had seen while I still held hope arrived. She and the nurse assembled in the room with a timid resident. The doctors stood at the foot of the bed, and the nurse stood to my left.

The nurse put her hand on my left leg and told Karim to put his on my right, as he had nearly five years earlier. I looked at the ceiling, pushed once, and hardly felt the baby's body pass out of mine. My mother gasped.

The doctors rushed him to the edge of the room, away from me, and the nurse began to massage my belly for the afterbirth. *Hardly any fluid at all,* she mumbled. And I was relieved.

My mother and sister left us alone. When the doctor brought him back to me, he was bundled into a hospital blanket, shrouded.

She gingerly peeled back the edges of the blanket, uncovering his face, like flower petals. I was as eager to see him as I had been to see my live baby. His face was small, pointed, and beautiful, in spite of the cleft lip. As she transferred him to me, she explained that the right side of his body was open, had never closed.

The bundle was light, like a nightmare in which your baby has disappeared. But he was there, and when I pulled back the blanket to see his body, his inky purple intestines were spilling out of his right side and sticking to the cotton. His entire body was the length of my forearm.

I opened his mouth, gently pushing down on his chin with my forefinger. There was no cleft in his palate. The roof of his mouth was whole and joined. He could have been fed without a tube.

His tiny tongue lay neatly behind his lower gums, pinkish gray and pointed like a cat's. He had faint eyebrows and eyelashes. His eyes would not open. His hands were gummy and curled, his brow furrowed.

My mother returned with a croissant and attempted to force bites into my mouth. I turned my head away, and golden flakes fell onto the receiving blanket enveloping the baby. I laughed hoarsely through tears. *Imagine when they do the autopsy. They'll find cafeteria croissant all over him.*

Karim took the baby from my arms, and my mother continued to feed me, both of us shivering with the laughter that comes too close on the heels of tears.

I held him one more time before the nurse came to take him. I kissed the tiny concentric swirl of fine hair on his cold, yielding forehead. And then he was gone.

Calendar of the Unexpected?

Catherine R. Squires

March 2001

My friend D from graduate school called to catch up with me in the winter of 2001. For some reason, I decided to go ahead and tell her: "I had a miscarriage."

"Oh—how far along *were* you?" she asked.

"Um, like eight or nine weeks," I stammered.

Then there was a pause, a silence, a hesitation on her end of the line.

"So it's not really a miscarriage, right? I mean—it wasn't really a baby yet, right?"

Though she was hundreds of miles away, I think she could sense my face reddening, or could hear my heart pounding and stomach twisting and gurgling in the effort to maintain a steady voice as I replied, "It was to me."

I remember sitting there, in the straight-backed dining room chair, looking out of the floor-to-ceiling windows of the home we were renting. It was a modernist retreat in a small wooded development with its own human-engineered lake near the banks of the Huron River. It had become my escape from the office, from well-meaning people, from the hospital. Looking out at the slim branches and trunks of the pine and birch and hemlock trees for hints of nuthatches, downy woodpeckers, and chickadees clinging to the bark, chirruping and honking in the gray light, on their quest for insects, keeping me company, keeping my mind occupied until Bryan returned from work on the winding river road.

* * *

A few weeks before D's phone call, I am lying on the exam table, cramping my neck to look over at the sonogram screen. The gynecologist taps on a gray circular form.

"Yes, see right there? Blighted ovum."

The gynecologist withdraws the sonogram wand and begins explaining what will happen next, over the next few days or possibly weeks, when my uterus expels the blighted ovum, the nondeveloping fertilized egg, the blob of cells that has ceased dividing and complexifying and growing. She pushes her stool away from the table, tosses her gloves into the waste can, and goes to the sink to begin washing her hands. All the while she continues explaining what will happen to the blighted ovum. It will detach from the blood-rich uterine wall, hormones will trigger contractions, and it will be pushed out, discarded, disposed.

I will bleed.

I will cramp.

I will feel pain.

I may need surgery if there are complications with the detachment.

I must look awful, because when the gynecologist finally finishes her recitation of the blighted ovum's scheduled demise and turns from the sink to look at me, she squints at me, like she's never seen a face like mine.

"Do you want to call someone?" she asks.

I have three more appointments with this gynecologist. At each one, I bring up how I am still feeling tired, having strangely long periods, and cannot get pregnant despite trying after the prescribed waiting period. I've read these are symptoms of possible thyroid issues, I say. She shrugs it off and suggests I am more likely depressed, that I might try anti-depressants, that I should keep trying to get pregnant despite how awful I feel, because I am getting closer to thirty, and it is harder after that decade begins.

My hair is falling out. I've gained a lot of weight. My periods have extended to almost two weeks of bleeding. I can't think straight, but I know it isn't depression. I try to remind her that it might have to do with my history of endometriosis, that I might have a hormonal imbalance.

She continues to dismiss what I describe, what I hypothesize about my body.

I change doctors.

I wait for six weeks to see a reproductive endocrinologist for a full hormonal workup.

I get many vials of blood taken for testing right after I turn in my paperwork.

After the blood draw, I meet the doctor. This doctor asks lots of questions, different questions, and he listens to my answers. He doesn't try to tell me what is wrong. He says we'll wait for the tests, and we'll know more.

I get a voice mail from him two days later.

"Catherine, your test results show a serious thyroid problem. You need to pick up a prescription as soon as possible. Please talk to my nurse for instructions if you can't reach me at this number."

It turns out that I have Hashimoto's disease and have had it for a long time. My body attacked its own thyroid gland, decimating its ability to make the crucial hormone. Hence the extended periods, hair loss, fatigue, weight gain, and infertility. The nurse tells me, "With your levels, there was no way you were getting pregnant!"

I am relieved. The miscarriage wasn't my fault, despite the accusation built within the word.

I begin my thyroid replacement medication.

I lose weight.

I take vitamins.

March 2002

I am pregnant with triplets. I am pregnant after my new doctor's interventions, which included a round of follicle stimulating hormones to "reboot" my ovaries after they went dormant from the thyroid nosedive. The doctor asks us if we want to "reduce" the number of embryos to reduce the risks carried by a multiple pregnancy. Bryan and I say, "No," simultaneously.

June 2002

I buy two books, the only two general-reader books I could find on high-risk, multiple pregnancies. I fold pages and put sticky notes in places. I take naps and a prenatal yoga class. I go swimming. I take prenatal vitamins. I make it past the first trimester. We celebrate by expanding the list of people we're willing to tell about the pregnancy. About triplets.

I eat a lot. I start eating meat again, after having been vegetarian since my college days. Near my birthday, we go to L and T's house for a July barbecue. I eat two and a half chicken breasts, pasta salad, and dessert. The next day I put on my maternity bathing suit and trudge across the street and up the hill to the public pool, but it is closed for repairs. I am shaking and sweating, and make my way back home and fall asleep on the couch.

* * *

I continue taking my qualitative methods workshop, a professional development module that meets twice a week. I tell the class I'm pregnant with triplets, excusing myself to go to the bathroom once again. "I'm constantly having to pee with these three," I joke, and my classmates smile at me. During the break, a few ask me how far along I am. One, a medical school professor, looks at me and says, "You don't look very big for that far along."

July 2002, Week 15

My mother and sister want to have a baby shower for me, and we drive to Evanston to visit and plan. I'm tired. I sleep in the car, and Bryan does all the driving. I don't feel comfortable behind the wheel; I feel like I can't reach the pedals and make enough room for my swollen belly, even though I'm not *that* big yet.

The second night we're there, Mom invites friends over for dinner, but I am tired and try to turn in early. My back also hurts, and I can't get comfortable on the queen-sized futon. Everyone's laughter in Mom's living room seems so loud. I want to ask them to be quiet, but instead I seethe in the dark until they leave.

We leave for home the next day, and as we head toward Sheridan Road, a crow flies into our car's windshield with a sick thump.

"Is it dead?" I ask Bryan. "Do you think it's dead?"

"I don't know. I hope not. Superstition, you know?"

July 29, 17½ Weeks

I wake up from an afternoon nap and go to the bathroom. I see a lot of blood on the toilet paper, and some substance I have never seen before. I rush to the phone to call the triage nurse, just like I was instructed by my high-risk obstetrician, Dr. Van de Ven.

"Do you see membranes?" the triage nurse asks me.

"What do they look like? There's blood and, I don't know, some kind of mucus?" I reply. I've never been pregnant with nonblighted ova, so I have no idea about these membranes.

"It's probably just spotting. Call back if you have cramping or contractions." She is blasé; she seems unconcerned, and like she has other patients with real problems to see. I say, "Okay," and hang up. I take a nap.

But when we sit down to eat dinner that evening, my body starts thrashing and churning out of control into early labor. Somehow Bryan is able to help me to the car, and we head to the hospital.

By the time we get to the hospital, my cervix is dilated two centimeters, flat and open. The amniotic sac of one of the three children is sagging into the opening. I had seen membranes that afternoon, after all. The attending physician goes to page my obstetrician.

Doctor Van de Ven comes in and asks us to discuss if we want to try to preserve the pregnancy or terminate it now, at seventeen weeks. He gives us a 10 percent chance of survival for the triplets. Bryan and I reply, "Preserve the pregnancy," simultaneously, before Dr. Van de Ven can even leave the room to give us time to talk in private.

* * *

Bryan holds my right hand as I lie on the gurney, moving through the hallways from triage to the room where I am being admitted. He only lets go when the night nurse wheels me through the doorway, lifts me, lays me in the bed, and tilts it to the prescribed degree.

One nurse stays by my left side at the head of the bed as it is slowly lowered, and grasps my hand. She is a solid, squat woman whose forearms could knead a hundred loaves of bread, then birth a calf, and stir a cast-iron kettle of porridge before sunrise. She is built to support life.

As the other nurse busies herself with wires and tubes and monitor settings, she keeps my left hand in hers. Bryan holds my right hand and looks into my eyes, smiling as much as he can. "It's going to be okay, Catherine." He repeats this over and over, rubbing his palm over the back of my hand. The other nurse turns to go, assuring Bryan on her way out the door that he can use the call button anytime.

The night nurse who was clutching my hand stays back a moment. Before releasing her grip, she embraces me, her thick arms easily bringing me to her warm torso. She whispers roughly in my ear, "I give you all my strength!"

Then, before I can thank her, she is out the door.

I never see that nurse again, but I feel her capacious chest and the firmness of her grasp on my left hand every day. I believe—I still believe—she transferred to me a gift.

* * *

This is what happens to you when your cervix opens up too early and you want to try to save the fetuses inside rather than terminate the pregnancy:

You get put on a bed tilted, head down, at five to ten degrees to take pressure off the cervix and ease the placenta back inside.

You get drugs to stop contractions.

You get a large IV shunt attached to your veins for antibiotics to stave off infections, and for fluids to stave off dehydration, which can bring on contractions.

You have a catheter inserted because you don't get up to pee.

You lie like this for many days until the doctors think there's a chance to place a cerclage in your cervix, to sew it up to everything inside.

So I lie upside down, on my back, hooked up to tubes and needles and monitors, for days. My world was officially off-kilter. I was literally on a different axis than the rest of the maternity wing, on another plane, like the diagrams of vectors moving through three-dimensional spaces in the math books Bryan used to prepare for teaching undergrads. We had to create our own map of this world, setting up a routine in an upside-down environment.

July 30

"I don't want to watch TV here," I declared, and Bryan agreed.

"Yes. We can use the VCR for a documentary or something," he suggested. And from there, we made spoken and unspoken rules for the hospital room that fit our physical confinement. I was hooked up to IVs and a catheter and could not get up. At all. He brought in sheets and pillows from home to settle into the reclining chair that converted to lie flat. It wasn't a true bed, but Bryan sat and slept every day and night in that contraption. From that chair, he would ask, "Do you want me to read some more tonight?" Another rule: we would read, meaning, Bryan read to me. He had checked out books from the library and bought some.

* * *

Looking back, I am really glad it was 2002. We didn't have smartphones, or Facebook, or Twitter, or Instagram. I'm pretty sure the hospital didn't even have Wi-Fi for patient rooms yet, because Bryan would take short breaks to go to his office—a good walk but not too far from the hospital—to check emails. I felt no need to update anyone on my status or to make choices about what to post online. I am eternally grateful I was pregnant before it was common for pregnant women to post selfies of their growing bellies, smiling triumphantly into the camera, proving their fertility and health. I was tortured enough by my memory of pictures on pregnancy books and magazines sitting on the bedside table in our townhouse, gathering dust while I lay in the hospital trying to beat 10 percent odds. Instead of making posts on a website or listserv, Bryan kept a small blue spiral notebook in his pocket, where he made notes of everything that happened during that first week in the hospital.

We were a team of two. There were few discussions about our situation: we were of a single mind in those days. "It's actually a relief," Bryan mused as he settled into his sleeping chair for the night. "I know exactly where I need to be and what I need to do, twenty-four hours a day. I just need to be here for you and the babies." He squeezed my hand and turned off the table lamp. The sun set and rose, nurses came and went. Bryan used the shower, shaved, and made quick trips to the cafeteria or home. But his steady support and love were the clear constant, my lodestar.

July 31

Dr. Van de Ven reported that my uterus had calmed down after two days of being on the incline and taking indomethacin, a uterine-calming drug. I had hoped as much, since I wasn't feeling the contractions anymore, but every breath or slight movement in my body had sparked fear that they were returning. But the amniotic sac for Baby A (they labeled multiples by letters in order from closest to cervix to farthest) was still sagging into my cervical opening.

"We're going to take you off this incline," Dr. Van de Ven notified us, explaining that "there's risk of blood pressure problems, and we've probably seen all the improvement we're gonna get with the gravity helping us." I wasn't sure if I should feel hopeful or discouraged by that, but I was glad to be back on level ground. I had an almost constant headache while on the sloped bed.

"And I want to try something," my doctor continued. His postdoctoral fellow arrived, wheeling an ultrasound machine in front of her. "There may be a way to close up that cervix."

Here's what they did:

Looking at my uterus with the ultrasound, they then used a syringe to pump water into the catheter, filling my bladder like a balloon. "See there?" Dr. Van de Ven pointed at the picture, while I felt the worst urge to go pee I'd ever had since I was in kindergarten. "See how the bladder pushes the cervix closed? If I can get a needle in there, I can run a stitch. We can do the cerclage." He looked at me and Bryan.

I looked at Bryan and saw he, like me, was nodding already.

"Okay, let's try it," I said.

I didn't realize until the nurses and administrator came with the paperwork that I had to sign waivers that I wouldn't sue the hospital if I or any of the triplets were harmed, or killed, by the procedure. I also didn't know they were going to use general anesthesia until that moment, because one thing I remembered from the books I'd bought on high-risk pregnancies was that a cerclage could be put in while you had a spinal block—numb from the waist down but awake. For some reason, I thought we'd be doing that, but it was general anesthesia instead. I was scared of going under general anesthesia but more scared of not trying to get my cervix closed. There was no way the babies would be "viable" at seventeen or eighteen or even nineteen weeks if I went into labor again, or infection set in, or whatever else could go wrong that I knew about. They would die. And I knew I would never want to get pregnant again. Never.

Hands shaking, I signed the papers.

By this time my mom had arrived. Bryan was there, and she was there. They stayed with me and walked with me as far as they could toward the surgery area. Bryan clasped my hand and smoothed my forehead as he walked alongside the gurney. Then he bent down to give me a kiss before they wheeled me away.

When they brought me into the OR, they put a hairnet on me, and hooked me up to a new set of monitors. Then the anesthesiologist started leading me through the procedure to knock me out. I had to keep my arms in a T position, and they strapped them down, just in case—of what I didn't really know. Then he fit a plastic mask over my face with a tube down my throat. I wasn't ready. The last thing I remember was trying to tell the anesthesiologist while gagging on the tube that I was not ready. But all he did was tell me to count backwards.

Then I woke up, puking into a plastic pan.

I was in a hallway or staging area, and it was dim. Bryan was holding my hand, looking down at me on the gurney. He had the saddest smile.

My throat was on fire with bile and the aggravation of the tube. I squawked, "What happened?"

Bryan squeezed my hand. "They tried sweetie, you did so well. They tried, but—the needle. There just wasn't enough room. The needle nicked the baby's sac."

One of our babies was dead.

I know Dr. Van de Ven said something to us before the nurses wheeled me back to the hospital room, but I didn't really hear him or understand. Bryan just kept telling me, "You did so good, Sweetie. You did so well." And I thought he was going to cry, but he didn't. All I could think was, "This is my fault. If only I had gone to triage and not let that nurse on the phone make me think I was being a hypochondriac. If only I had taken more naps, or not taken the class, or not tried to walk to the pool. If I had known about membranes. If only I had done some small or large or insignificant thing differently," I railed at myself, silently, tears flowing, "our babies wouldn't be in danger. All of them would be alive. And we would be at home. Safe."

*   *   *

Sometime that night, Dr. Van de Ven came by and asked us again if we wanted to continue trying to save the other two babies. It was inevitable that my body would reject the dead body, and the risk of infection was high. It was most likely that once my uterus started to expel the dead fetus, all three would come out. "I can't even give you a percentage, what the chances are, that they could stay inside," he said, sounding like he had been crying. His eyes were usually so bright, but their blue was dulled, tired.

Somehow, in that moment that I knew our babies would make it. I recalled a dream I had, of being on our big new bed at home, with a nursing pillow and two babies. Not three, two. I remembered being upset by that dream, but now it was something to cling to.

We told Dr. Van de Ven, as before, that we wanted to try to preserve the pregnancy.

August 1

Bryan resumed reading to me. I was taken off the catheter, and Dr. Van de Ven allowed me a trip or two to the bathroom each day, and a shower. I hadn't showered for days. I smelled of medicine and urine and saline. I cried as the warm water cascaded over my shaking shoulders and quaking legs. My belly looked pitifully small and inadequate. But then I breathed in deep and straightened up.

"Mom, I need you to cut my hair," I declared after the shower. Mom was with me while Bryan took a break and checked in at home with our bills and other mundane things.

Mom was puzzled. "Are you sure?"

"Yes." I asked the nurse for some scissors, but all she would give us were the safety scissors for cutting off bandages, not office scissors even. I didn't care.

She repeated her question: "Are you sure you want me to cut your hair, with these?"

"Yes, Mom." And with some nervous laughter, she began.

I had been growing my hair out when I got pregnant. I imagined throwing my hair up into braids, or a bun, or a ponytail before changing diapers or pushing a triple stroller for a power walk to the grocery store. Nothing was going to be like I imagined, and I needed to make a mark to make that clear. Confined to the hospital room, cutting my hair was one thing I could control and could change easily. And my mom was the only one I wanted to do it for me. I felt relief as each curl fell to the floor.

August 4

I never saw the solid, comforting nurse who brought me into the hospital the first night. But I remembered her and her generosity at the moment I met an intern I'd never met before. At that moment, I was at the beginning phase of having to expel my dead son from my body. The intern's body language and voice had the opposite effect of the solid nurse's presence, and the intern's stance might have ended my time in the hospital with three deaths rather than one, because when she looked at me, in my contraction pain and panic, she asked me this: "Do you mind giving birth right here?"

I looked at her and saw contempt with a smidgen of pity in her green eyes peering at me through fashionable glasses. She blew a stray piece of brownish-blond lanky hair away from her eyes, as if to see this strange specimen more clearly. All I could do was stammer, "I guess so."

The intern didn't offer to find my husband, or my doctor, or the postdoctoral fellow who was assisting Dr. Van de Ven with my case. She just stood there looking down at me while the nurses came to try to get me all the way onto the bed. She didn't lift a finger or move an inch to assist them or me, didn't go get a sterile bed pad, or wash her hands or anything. She just watched me until she was pushed out of the way by my husband, who miraculously returned soon, followed by the appearance of the postdoc. Like Athena from Zeus's head, the postdoc sprang out of nowhere into wise action. I couldn't see the intern's reaction to the postdoc's order to "Book a surgical suite now. Dr. Van de Ven is on his way up." The postdoc was going to get me to the surgery to give my babies a chance to live, not just expelled along with their dead brother's body.

Dr. Van de Ven had a plan, though he hadn't shared it with me and Bryan yet. Unbeknownst to us, he had been doing research. He found reports from an Arab doctor in the Emirates or somewhere in that part of the world, who had preserved a twin after its sibling had been born preterm. The key was leaving the placenta inside, on the other side of the cervical canal, tricking my body into thinking it wasn't time for more contractions to expel the other two placental sacs. Not time for gestation to be over. The time to expel everything and start the nurturance phase outside of the womb had not yet come. Eventually, my cervix started to close down, and we tried a second cerclage. It worked.

* * *

Not long ago, the news was full of headlines about Serena Williams's story of almost dying after giving birth. The hospital staff wouldn't believe her when she described her deadly health condition, which was worsening postdelivery. They greeted her with suspicion rather than care. When I think about Williams's story, and when I see statistics that the rate of black maternal death is 243 percent higher than white maternal death, I can't help but wonder if race played any role in that intern's disdain for me the day my son was stillborn. I think about the gynecologist who was perfectly fine ignoring my concerns about thyroid symptoms. I'll never know if race played a role, but it is not outside the realm of possibility. Studies do show that health workers regularly dismiss or minimize black patients' concerns, minimize their pain, and dismiss claims of trauma. If a superstar like Serena Williams, pregnant in a private hospital where she and her husband paid to get special treatment, can't get nurses to treat her with respect, to acknowledge that she is feeling something wrong in her body and give her care that she needs, what can the rest of us expect?

October 1, 28 Weeks, 10 p.m.

After two months of bed rest with biweekly visits from a nurse, the contractions begin again.

Bryan drives me to triage, as we are instructed. We tell them I am Dr. Van de Ven's patient, and about the early labor. But the doctor assigned to us doesn't admit me.

"We have to be sure that the contractions are getting closer together. You can lay down in there, and we'll time them and take a look at the cerclage."

"Did you talk to Dr. Van de Ven?" I ask. The doctor just replies, "Hospital admission rules. I'll get a nurse to set you up to rest in there."

I am flummoxed. How can they do this? Aren't we supposed to be on some sort of list, some sort of emergency list of people who have dangerous pregnancies? I had read in my books that I should be getting a dose of magnesium sulfate to pacify all of my muscles, the uterus especially. Get shots of steroids to strengthen the babies' lungs, in case the magnesium sulfate treatment doesn't have the desired effect. There are things to be done, but instead we are ushered into a side room, where a bunch of spare gurneys are sitting under half-dimmed lights. Bryan helps me get up on the metal gurney and puts a blanket over me and the uterine monitor strapped to my belly. It is 11:00 p.m.

October 2, 28 Weeks and 1 Day, 2 a.m.

The doctor returns. She checks my uterine monitor and the readouts. "We're going to admit you."

I get the magnesium sulfate and begin to float between worlds. I don't even feel the pneumatic needles pushing into my thigh, delivering the steroids for the twins' underdeveloped lungs.

I dream constantly. At one point, on one day, I tell a friend who's come to sit with me so Bryan can take a break, "Write this down for me." What I say is unintelligible to her, because she didn't write it. But I remember saying, "I can see my son and daughter in my arms. They will be okay."

October 3, 28 Weeks, 2 Days

I am allowed to have a sponge bath to get the heavy metallic smell off my body. I luxuriate with each sweep of the washcloth the nurse assists me with, even though I am naked in front of someone I don't know. I don't care. I can feel the babies moving inside me.

October 4, 28 Weeks, 3 Days: Birth Day

I wake up feeling fluid between my legs. It isn't urine or blood or membranes, just clear.

My water has broken.

A new doctor I haven't met before brings an ultrasound machine to check the fluid levels and says it's Baby A's sac ("Baby A is Will, my son," I think in my head, cross with her). She says that it is leaking, but my uterus is not contracting, so as long as the fluid stays at a sufficient level, we're okay.

Two hours later, Dr. Van de Ven visits and declares, "Today is the day. Those babies are coming out."

Twenty-eight and a half weeks. My babies are being delivered two months early. I wanted to get to thirty-two weeks, at least.

Dr. Van de Ven explains that because he left the placenta in to preserve the pregnancy, to trick my body into waiting, the placenta is now an infection risk. With the punctured sac, Will could get an infection that would also spread to me and Helena.

October 4 would be their birthday.

October 4, 2 p.m.

I prepare myself for the spinal block, curling myself inward and pushing my spine toward the anesthesiologist's needle, inviting it to find an easy slot between my vertebrae.

"You made that easy!" He raises his eyebrows and peers at me as the nurse helps me lie back onto the gurney.

"I've had practice," I manage to joke. The cerclage at eighteen and a half weeks had been set with only a spinal block.

Bryan is allowed in as soon the spinal block starts taking effect. He has to wear a hairnet and a surgical gown, but they don't make him wear a mask. "Our babies are coming today, Sweetie. You did so good." He squeezes my hand, then stands where I can see him, but not in the way of the doctors who file in and take positions on the other side of the surgical drape. I can't see what they are doing, but I can see Dr. Van de Ven's blue eyes, and I relax as much as I can.

I feel a tugging sensation in my lower body and back as they cut into my uterus and begin moving things around to bring the babies out.

Will is first. He is so small. I lose my breath at how small he is. I can't really see his eyes, but I can hear the start of a faint wail. Then he is taken away by the nurse for the Apgar test, the test that will determine what medical interventions will be started right away, and what will wait for the neonatal intensive care unit. But I hear breath from him, if not the classic infant cry.

Helena is next. She is bigger, just slightly, and her skin is so much redder than her brother's. Dr. Van de Ven holds her up over the curtain a little longer. "Helena," I whisper up at Bryan, tears coming down my face. Then she is gone.

"Go with them," I urge Bryan. "Please—I don't want them to be alone."

Bryan looks torn. "I want you to go with them," I repeat. And he follows their trail to the heated stations where the tests are happening.

In a few minutes, he reports back.

"They're both over two pounds! They're not going to intubate them, they think."

A miracle. The steroids have worked.

"They're taking them to the NICU now." Bryan puts his hand on my forehead.

"Go with them," I manage to choke.

"Are you sure?"

"Yes. Be with our babies." And he goes with Dr. Van de Ven, while his surgical residents start the task of reconstructing my abdomen.

The residents are a chatty bunch, talking with each other on the other side of the drape, putting their hands inside my body, as if I can't hear them. They wear plastic eyeshades and paper masks over their mouths, and with the glare it is hard for me to see their eyes. The residents stand, talking to each other, just three figures in blue surgical scrubs, every so often raising their bloody, gloved hands above my stomach.

October 4, Evening

"Here comes Mom," I hear the nurse call ahead of my gurney as she opens the security doors to the NICU. Bryan is there. The twins are placed on my chest, above my sutured belly. I am crying, "Oh, Sweeties! Mommy is here! Mommy is here! I am so glad to see you!" They are so light, I can hardly believe these are the creatures who kicked my ribs and elbowed my organs for the past two months.

Blighted

Elsa Valmidiano

Blight, noun.

1 Any of numerous plant diseases resulting in sudden conspicuous wilting and dying of affected parts, especially young, growing tissues.
2 The condition or causative agent, such as a bacterium, fungus, or virus, that results in blight.
3 An agent or action that harms or ruins the value or success of something.
4 A condition or result of harmful or ruinous action.

A wand, and not a magical one, is inserted into my vagina to inspect the fetal pole that Husband and I should've seen on the ultrasound screen, but there is nothing but an empty misshapen circle. In medical terms, there's a sac and placenta but nothing else. Doctor's face immediately falls from a hopeful smile to furrowed brows. As Doctor and I both search the screen for that much-anticipated gummy bear that so many expectant mothers are dying to see, Husband instead notices the worried look painted across Doctor's face. He knew something was wrong before I did.

"There is a placenta and sac but no fetal pole . . . Anembryonic pregnancy . . . We should've seen a fetal pole by now at eleven weeks . . . When did you say your last period was, and you haven't had any spotting or bleeding since then?"

These phrases stumble in my head as *the* answer. The unequivocal answer. It wasn't so much a death sentence. More so, it was an incomplete sentence. *Incomplete.* It did not grow. It ended abruptly. Somewhere. The sperm met the egg, but that was it. A sac and placenta continued to grow giving way to a deceptive belly that held absolutely nothing but maybe a few bits and pieces of a fertilized egg.

Doctor had also called it "blighted ovum." The fertilized egg had blighted. Deteriorated. Due to a bad egg. Or bad sperm. It hadn't been my fault. The fertilized egg decided on its own to disintegrate. But wasn't it *my* egg? Did not the egg belong to *my* body? A product of my own body? It appears rebellion starts not just young, but when one simply comes into being, even for ten measly minutes of being.

Blighted vine of my being.

How and when did it make up its own mind to end its own beginning? Or maybe my body simply rejected it for being bad. A bad egg. A blighted egg. It never even got to the stage of being a naughty him or her.

I had been under the misconception that miscarriages strictly took place under the spontaneous expulsion of an embryo or fetus. I had no idea that a miscarriage could also result from a fertilized egg that never develops, though in my case, the cells destined to become the placenta and membranes continued to develop despite the absence of an embryo. For ten weeks, my slightly bulging belly gave me the impression that I was pregnant, when in fact, I was simply carrying an empty home.

Five minutes later, hospital gown tossed into the basket, and clothes back on, I asked with calm urgency, "What now? Should I wait to miscarry?"

"Seeing how far along you are, I wouldn't suggest it. You could get an infection. You could hemorrhage. You'd need a D&C."

"Can we schedule one soon?"

"I'd still need to take blood tests to check your hCG levels, to see if they will drop. You may miscarry within the week."

But I knew I wasn't going to ever miscarry, whatever that meant. Miscarry. The life within me had obviously ended, and yet I was still holding its fully furnished home with a fully stocked fridge, but no nine-month tenant to house and feed. I had a strong intuition that whatever was inside of me was going to hold on.

"I'll have to check your hCG levels first," Doctor repeated.

I wanted it out then and there, but I suppose she just had been following standard operating procedure.

"I'll need two blood tests, forty-eight hours apart."

We hadn't told many people about me being pregnant, having been prepared for a worst-case scenario, but as I reached the tenth week with no sign of miscarrying, I thought we were in the clear, so we enthusiastically told a few more people about the pregnancy a few days leading up to the ultrasound.

But on the day of the ultrasound, after we found out, we wasted no time sending out texts as soon as we arrived home.

I drafted the text, and Husband copied it to every one of his friends and family. I ticked each one off my own small list when the text was sent. We wasted no tears or time with anyone. It wasn't news we wanted to deliver, but we delivered it promptly like ripping off a Band-Aid.

Husband and I went for the first test on Saturday morning. Then the follow-up on Monday morning.

"Is it okay if we head out of town as we had originally planned, or should we cancel our plans?" I asked Nurse.

Nurse replied, "You can head out of town as long as you can drive back to Oakland immediately if you start miscarrying."

"We'll be four hours away."

Nurse paused. "Four hours is not bad."

"I'll make sure that a hospital is close by."

Actually, I never did. I assumed there would be a hospital in the area. We were in California after all.

Blighted, adjective.

   1 Anything that mars or prevents growth or prosperity.

On our first stop, Husband and I had gone strawberry picking. The fields stretched before us, the beach not far from where my long hair whipped wildly in the wind. While bending down to pick the reddest, juiciest strawberries, I remembered a *tita* who once told me that fruits were the ripened ovaries of a plant, so imagine a field of ovaries, hanging red, ripe, and low, innocently waiting to be plucked by our greedy hands, or blighted by the birds ready to swoop up and devour.

The next few days consisted of hiking, biking, and kayaking in a quaint beach town on the Central Coast. It had been our first-year wedding anniversary, and this would've been our way of celebrating not only our anniversary but the promise of a new little one. On our second day there, Doctor confirmed my hCG levels remained high and steady as if I were twelve weeks pregnant, despite the ultrasound evidence of no fetus. She figured, as well as I, that the possibility of miscarrying on my own was almost nil. She scheduled a D&C for that Friday.

The week prior, Husband and I had made love, as if the three of us were connected through our intimacy, when it had been unknowingly the two of us, beckoning at a vacant hearth. Now, we did not make love on this anniversary but simply held each other in the dark, waiting for Friday.

By the fourth day of our vacation, there were still no signs of miscarrying. Every trip to the bathroom, I'd search for that sign of dropping. I'd find nothing. As I predicted, my body would hold on.

The night before the procedure, I received a call from my mother. She left a short voice mail with her condolences. I refused to take the call, as my mother's words are tears themselves, and it is my situation that makes us both remember her miscarriage. It was the miscarriage before me. What I call a true miscarriage. Her body had expelled my older sibling into the toilet, which is how I thought all miscarriages occurred. She had been in her first trimester, maybe at the end. Her body had expelled a gray mass of what was to be her child. My father thought it had been a boy. My mother thought it had been her fault. She blamed herself, as my two older siblings were just recovering from the measles then, and she blamed herself for having been in contact with sick children during her early pregnancy. But they were her children who needed her, who needed to be taken care of.

She could not save the gray mass of what was to be her child, so she prayed over the toilet before flushing him/her down. She went in for a D&C and then immediately went on maternity leave, as that was the policy of the Philippines then. Following miscarriage or birth, that's what a woman did. A woman went on maternity leave. Where are those laws in my parents' adopted country? My mother received condolences from people at work, although she felt the condolences were insincere and simply standard operating procedure. She didn't need condolences. Neither did I.

Like my mother, I decided to tell my job, declaring my own kind of maternity leave, not because I necessarily wanted to, but because the probable risk of experiencing bright-red bleeding afterward might require necessary recovery time. I wasn't afraid to give myself that time. Also, I could. I knew not very many women could.

I think of what the D&C looked like for my mother in 1976. There were no machine vacuum aspirators then. Just metal instruments that scooped and scraped. There were never machine vacuum aspirators in the Philippines. To this day, they at most have manual vacuum aspirators that remind me of cheap plastic tubes used for pesticide spray. Abortion is illegal in the Philippines, which in turn makes the same advanced medical technology to surgically complete miscarriages also illegal.

As an American, I consider myself lucky. As a Filipina living in California, I consider myself very lucky.

When I think of my mother, I think, *Now we have something in common.*

Blight, verb.

   1 To cause to wither or decay; blast.
   2 To destroy; ruin; frustrate.

Friday arrives. I lie on my side in a hospital gown as Nurse injects a serum at the base of my back to help with cramping later. I am wearing a black-and-white mini dress with flowers and am told to undress only from the waist down. Since I'm wearing a mini dress, I hike the hem to my waist and cover the bottom half of myself with the gown. Suddenly I'm an *aswang*. Mythical creature of my childhood, usually a vampire seductress whose top half would dislodge from her bottom half at the waist, taking flight with her long dragon wings, searching for an innocent pregnant woman to slither her tongue and eat the woman's unborn child. Had my body eaten my own child by reabsorbing it back into itself?

"Will the shot hurt?" I ask Nurse. She says it feels like a tetanus shot. I think of a long epidural needle going in, but it's not an epidural. It's a quick, heavy pinch. I suppose some women become *aswang* during childbirth, losing the feeling in their legs with the help of an epidural, their bottom halves dislodging while their torso takes flight in some part of their mind far away.

Husband stands in the room, not knowing what to do. I ask him to touch me. "Put your hand on my shoulder." He complies. The weight of his hand on my shoulder doesn't comfort me but instead feels patronizing, and I want to cry because of it. I feel disappointed, not for the failed pregnancy, but that I disappointed everyone in having to tell them that it had failed.

Husband rubs my arm as Nurse instructs me to continue lying on my side while the shot takes effect. I hold in my tears as I focus on the numbers of a machine next to me. I don't know what the machine is for, but it's not for the procedure. Everything that will be used—metal instruments and vacuum—is covered with heavy white tissue paper on a tray table a few feet away. I point to it and tell Husband, "There it all is." He responds, "I don't want to know."

Would he have traded places with me? Did he love me that much that he would've in a heartbeat?

I ignore the diagrams that decorate every gynecologist's office, the diagrams that paint sex simply as a scientific event and phenomenon for procreation and existence. The diagrams of a man's and woman's reproductive anatomies—the picture of a vagina and uterus full-blown to reveal details: stages of ovulation, stages of pregnancy, the layers of tissues surrounding the entrance of the vagina, while the picture of a penis and scrotum full-blown to reveal details: stages of spermatogenesis, the layers beneath the shaft, while there I was on the doctor's table, feet cold, and my half-naked body barely covered by the usual flimsy hospital gown, which failed to keep me warm. I felt, once again, like a lab rat.

The mere idea of sexual enjoyment seemed a farce, as the diagrams depicted human life as nothing but a long visual equation.

Emotions seemed to have no place in a doctor's office with its white antiseptic walls, blasting air conditioner, and the tissue paper on the table, which crunched and wrinkled as a patient uncomfortably shifted her weight.

Where and what was love, when gynecological procedures just boiled down to this one moment when a woman lies down on a doctor's table with feet elevated on stirrups.

Before Doctor instructs Husband to leave and wait in the waiting room, she asks if I want Valium or painkillers. I say no. I'm afraid it will make me nauseous. "I had an abortion, a D&E, almost twenty years ago, and I remember how the pills made me sick. I'd rather not be nauseous during and after this."

At first I falter and say "ten years" before declaring it twenty. Or maybe it was fifteen. My math skills had become inoperative despite the arresting memory of the abortion invariably time-stamped in my brain. But the sum didn't matter. Doctor didn't care how long it had been, as I noticed an expression of relief wash over her face as she learned the procedure wasn't so unfamiliar to me as she had originally thought.

"It won't be as quick as the last time, but should take at most ten to fifteen minutes," she says.

It'll be like coming home after twenty years, I think. Well, not exactly, but I knew what she meant, and I felt relieved that it wasn't awkward or shocking for me to say, and for her to hear, "I had an abortion, a D&E, almost twenty years ago." There isn't any need to justify to her why I had an abortion at twenty. Doctor doesn't need that explanation, but I'm sure the information is helpful.

At twenty, I was in an abusive relationship. I had no insurance then and covered the abortion through cash I pulled that very afternoon from the campus ATM. But there is no reason why that information is relevant now. I was in her office. I was in her office on her table for a much-needed procedure. There is no reason to defend why I needed to be in her office. Or why I needed to be in another office twenty years ago. Abortion is abortion. Miscarriage is miscarriage. Should it make any difference what we call it, especially in this moment while I'm lying half-naked on top of a table with knees spread?

Doctor asks if I want to listen to music during the procedure. I say, "No. I'll just go to my happy place."

"Do you want me to talk you through it?"

"Yes, please."

Before electing to undergo the D&C, my options were general anesthesia or local. If I had chosen general, Doctor would have had to refer me to another doctor at a hospital, as she doesn't administer general at her small clinic. But I wanted her to perform the D&C. I didn't want another doctor. I elected local anesthesia, but mostly because I'm the type of person that if I could have open-heart surgery completely awake and aware, I'd do it. I couldn't go without knowing what was being done to my body. I would need to know.

She injects the local anesthesia at my cervix, the narrow necklike passage connecting the vagina and uterus. What a small but significant passage between such continents that male politicians love having dominion over. The next infinite minute feels like a very long pap smear. She warns me of the sound of a vacuum before she turns it on. It doesn't scare me. *I am an old hat at this,* I think to myself in a strangely proud way. I hear the vacuum, and then there is endless tugging accompanied by her apologies, which suddenly makes me think of being reclined in a dentist's chair. It suddenly occurs to me why abortions have been analogized to dental visits. It occurs to me, *I am lucky.*

Almost ten years before this moment, I had worked at an organization in my motherland, the Philippines, which medically assisted women in the safe completion of dangerous and clandestine self-induced abortions. To save hospitals from criminal liability, medical records listed "spontaneous abortion" as the cause, while omitting the mention of catheters or perforations found upon admittance. I think of all the ways I have seen women accomplish one goal where, to this day, they are seen as criminal. I think of *hilot,* massaging the baby out with fists, *makabuhay* leaves boiled like tea, how we all will make choices even when the alley is dark and scary with coat hangers, catheters, bamboo sticks, toothpaste, and black-market Cytotec pills, or when the alley has a light on the other side with low humming machines, fresh surgical gloves, anesthesia, and antibiotics. The darkness or light of the alley never stopped women. And I remember, *I am lucky.*

The vacuum continues. The tugging continues. My left hand firmly grips my belly. My right hand firmly grips my right thigh. Nurse kindly reminds me to breathe, even though I'd rather hold my breath. I wonder why breathing is so important when holding one's breath never felt so necessary. I breathe because it feels like a command, but I'd rather not breathe. I breathe deep, simply to impress Nurse. Deep. Ten minutes feels like ten hours. I am wondering when I'll be able to relax. I'm wondering when the instruments will slide out of me. I'm waiting for that slide of relief. I remind myself, *I am lucky. I am lucky.*

For a moment, my mind unplugs from my body, and I become a sports commentator giving a play-by-play while also happening to feel her same acute pain. How is it that women can disengage from their bodies as if we are stadiums hosting a massive football game with thousands of fans cheering or booing in the stands for a clear winner. Our bodies—venues to be owned by corporate sponsors and not ourselves.

"You're doing great," Doctor reassures me.

"Thanks," I tell her, though I realize how weird that sounds immediately after I've said it.

As Doctor continues to tug and extract, I manage to relive my abortion of nearly twenty years ago. I recall how much more devastated I had felt about my abortion than I had for this miscarriage. Maybe because it had been the first pregnancy at such a young age, a pregnancy I wished hadn't existed at all. With this anembryonic pregnancy, friends and family wanted me to talk, almost expected me to, while it was clear abortion wasn't something you were supposed to talk about at all, as if the pregnancy meant less because it was unwanted. It seemed those around me generally held less compassion over abortion than they did over miscarriage, even though both can be safely completed by vacuum aspiration. While both continue to be associated with stigma and shame, it was clear that the end of one pregnancy could be judged more egregiously than the other, depending on the judge, as first-degree murder, while the other as involuntary manslaughter. You see how one can expect to meet either punishment or pardon.

I stare at the corner of the ceiling, falling into my happy place to distract me from the tugging and whirring. It isn't really a happy place, but the place where my mind rests to figure out math problems, what is right, what is wrong, what is what. *I blight it—My body blights it—It blighted—I—My body—It—Blight—What—Whom—By whom—Am I my body and is this not a part of me?*

"Without the activists who have fought and continue to fight for the continued legalization of abortion, the medical research and technology to advance procedures such as D&E and D&C would not be in existence today," I say as a keynote speaker standing at some misplaced podium in my mind addressing a judgmental faceless audience.

It matters. And then it doesn't, as I imagine other women, other mothers, others who believe in the sanctity of life want to tell me what happened to me but do not bother to listen.

My mind snaps back to present as the speculum is slid out of me. Finally. Doctor apologizes as she needs to do one more ultrasound to see if she got everything. "Do what you need to do. I understand." I can't remember if I say that or just think it. With the not-so-magical wand back in, she apologizes again as she has to go back in one more time for two more minutes, sliding a warm speculum in, except the metal feels hot, not warm. I gasp a little.

"Sorry," she says. "I didn't realize it was going to be warmer than usual."

A few more minutes. Maybe three.

And then I'm done. She's done. She snaps her gloves off.

"How does everything look?" I say. I need to know. Honestly.

"Everything looks good. You did great," she says triumphantly. And I believe her.

In the Month of August

Kao Kalia Yang

It begins with a love story.

I can still see that day, fresh in my memory as a favorite scene in a beloved movie. I'm standing at the pulpit of a church in a white button-up shirt, tucked into dress pants. There's a big skylight at the roof of the high ceiling. The early spring sunshine washes over me from the high window. The dust particles glitter and fly among the people in the big room, waiting for my words. My words, small words born from a tight throat, grow large in the power of the microphone before me.

He is a young man, but he is already balding. A wealthy white boy from the gentle suburbs of the cities, he sits in the room, perfectly straight. His big hands, long, fine fingers, rest casually in his lap. He looks at me, at first with the distant look of mere curiosity, and then growing interest. His nose is crooked. His face, full of facial hair, is soft, no hard bones jutting out, just round curves running through. It is not until he smiles at the end of my talk that I see the handsome in his face, a face that is common in this part of the country, until I notice the sparkle in his gaze.

One day, months later, we go on a walk together. We hold hands. My head barely clears his shoulders. The air is heavy with the growth of summer. The sky is moody. A warm wind blows the hair off my shoulder. With each step we take, the wind picks up. The clouds roll in, and the sky looks like a garage door shutting from the far distance. There is a rumble from the belly of the heavy clouds, a hungry snarl for food, for sustenance, for satisfaction. Soon, lightning is flashing across the gray. The sun is gone. The weather has turned. Rainfall, heavy and strong. I tighten my hold on his hand. He is pulling me. We are running through the storm. There is nowhere to hide. We end up hiding in ourselves and each other because the world has become a wet place, full of wild winds, and we are still young and fearless.

When at last we get home, after we've dried ourselves, we laugh from the adrenaline of our flight in the gray. We know we've flirted with danger, and each other. We thought then that we knew how dangerous life could be. We believed that somehow we were braver together than apart.

On August 6, 2011, we stood in front of our family and our friends, we extended our wrists in the fashion of my people, and we received the blessings of those who loved us and wished us well. White cotton strings filled our wrists and anchored us to each other in marriage.

I found myself in a shared life, planning a shared future. Late at night, when the world had grown quiet and the busy of the day had dimmed, we both looked out our bedroom window, a square full of sky, starlight and moonlight mingling, airplanes and shooting stars shifting across the high heavens. We talked of the future. We whispered of babies. There in that talk, without our knowing, we planted our first seeds of grief together.

August 2012 was hot. The tall grass fields across the Minnesota prairie were thirsty, drying at their tips, golden in the hot sun like fields of wheat. The earth was cracked in places, thirsty for rain. Big grasshoppers flew, their wings widespread across the fields of tall grass. Beneath the sun, they resembled butterflies.

My husband and I were happy about our first pregnancy. We got the best prenatal care we knew how to get from his graduate student health care at the university. We kept all our appointments at the midwives' clinic in the big hospital downtown. We walked often. We made sure that I ate healthy foods. I took the prenatal vitamins—especially the folic acid—despite the fact that I struggled to swallow the big pills down.

I watched as my belly began to grow round. At nineteen weeks, my regular clothes no longer fit. I invested in yoga pants and maternity tights. I engaged in conversation about how there was no maternity wear for women under five feet, and I laughed. It was with great excitement that I scheduled my first ultrasound.

I scheduled the appointment for a weekday. I took the first available appointment of the morning, eight fifteen. Outside, the late-summer sun was already beginning its work. I felt the hot rays on the back of my neck, heating up my hair. In the hospital parking ramp, the cement held on to the coolness of the night. There were parking spaces galore that morning. I pointed to the plethora of excellent spaces, close to the elevators. Together, my husband and I rejoiced, believing that the available parking spaces were just one more blessing in a world full of them.

We held hands as we walked to the OB testing unit. There was a lightness to my step that I hadn't felt in months. My husband held my hand firmly in his warm one. Occasionally, I touched my belly with my free hand.

If I could live in that moment of sunshine, make that walking ramp longer, miles and miles longer than it actually was, kept my girlish spirits high, I would, but alas I couldn't.

In the dim ultrasound room, I rested on the bed, my dress high up on my chest, the hill of my stomach wet with warm gel. My husband sat beside me in a chair. He continued holding one of my hands, playing with my fingers. We watched as the screen flickered on with the press of a button. I saw the spine of my baby, curved in a ball, turned toward the dark of my belly. The technician pressed a few more buttons. She moved the scanner from one side of my stomach to the other, up and down. I felt sleepy and content.

She asked, "Are you sure that your baby is nineteen weeks?"

Both my husband and I answered softly, caught in our dream spaces, "Yes."

The technician was quiet, too. She did more measurements. She shifted in her chair. She got up.

She said in a bare whisper, "Excuse me."

She left the room, closing the door firmly behind her.

The screen was still on. I patted my stomach with light fingers. I wanted my baby to wake up, to move, to turn around, to turn toward me. I laughed at myself: every direction the baby could possibly turn would be toward me. I patted my stomach some more.

I said, "Baby, wake up, Mommy and Daddy want to see you, wake up. *Me ab sawv os koj niam thiab koj txiv xav pom koj.*"

The door to the room opened with no warning. Two doctors came in. One was an older woman.

She said, "I'm Dr. Lupo," perhaps only in a regular voice, but somehow it dispelled the mood of the room.

The second woman, much younger, extended her hand to my husband. I don't remember her name, but she must have said it. I remember only that she was a resident. I remember only the feel of her hand on my left foot. Her hands were cool. She squeezed lightly.

Dr. Lupo walked to the screen. The young woman kept her hand on my left foot. Dr. Lupo straightened her mouth. She tapped the keys a few times. She turned toward me. She was an actor in a play. Her movements had been directed. Her words were pre-written.

She said, "I'm sorry. Your baby is dead."

The curtains closed on me.

My world was dark.

I listened for applause that did not come.

We were three days from our first anniversary; it was August 3, 2012, when Baby Jules was pronounced dead inside of me.

My husband and I were presented with two choices. We could go home and wait for the baby to abort naturally, or we could go to the labor and delivery unit, and the doctors could induce labor.

My hands kept shaking on my belly. They moved like butterfly wings.

We called our parents. My husband cried so much he couldn't speak. I took the phone from him.

I said, "We are at the hospital. The baby is dead."

I couldn't get more words out. The calls died in my hands one by one.

When there was no one else to call, my shaking hands returned to my belly. I kept thinking: You fan a fire into life, Kalia, you fan a fire into life.

The tears welled up inside of me and exploded in my throat.

We decided on option two.

They induced me.

The doctors who visited and the nurses in labor and delivery told me that the baby would come by nightfall.

By the time evening had settled heavy and thick over the city, they told me the baby would come by morning.

In the dark of the night, I heard the screams of women in pain. I heard the cries of their babies being born. I turned from the walls toward the one window in the room.

The window overlooked a church. There was a round, stained-glass window high on the church that depicted a figure of a man on his knees, his head bowed. I knew who the man was, although I did not belong to the Christian tradition. When I was a child and I was scared in the dark, I used to imagine the arms of my ancestors around me, holding me safe in the circle of their love. I listened for the quiet comfort of those who'd come before me, but all I heard was the hum of the machines around me. I sat still and quiet through the stretch of the long night, waiting for day to emerge from the far eastern sky. I felt the weight of sorrow grow inside of me, centering, deep and low in my belly. I curled on the bed in absent pain.

My husband sat beside me in a chair. He had his head down, although I knew he was not asleep. I heard his cries each time a baby was born somewhere on the ward. He gave voice to the cries choking my throat.

Morning came in slowly, slow gray cutting into the folds of night, then pink sunlight entered the room.

The early morning nurses and the doctors visited.

They said, "Not yet?"

We shook our heads. They put more medication inside of me.

It was noon. I could tell because there were no shadows in the room. Just the shine of sun from the window, the wash of light from the fluorescent bulbs overhead.

I wanted to go to the bathroom. My husband helped me up from the bed. He held my hand, and we walked to the bathroom, much as we had on numerous other occasions, inside the safety of walls, within the hold of nature. He might have even swung our hands—as was his habit. Inside the bathroom, our walk was done. We stood side by side. I looked at his shoulder. He closed the door. For a moment, he held me in his arms, and the world was very far away.

He said into my hair, "You have to let go."

My arms fell from around him.

I felt something drop in my belly, the weight I had been harboring deep inside of me, the child we had made but could not keep.

The baby came . . . a little boy, mouth opened like a little bird, a little boy who looked like a version of me, eyes closed, skin translucent, a little boy who weighed nothing in my arms—despite the weight I had felt with him inside of me, the weight of life, the weight of hope, the weight of humanity, the gravity of my little love story—his body was more light than anything else it could have ever been.

That autumn, we took long walks. I thought I should sit down and write. I couldn't. The emptiness was vast inside of me. I felt hollow as the wind shifted and the weather turned. The flowers I loved started to die, one by one. The cold grew inside of me until I wished I could melt away. The contradictions in what I felt and what I wanted were not lost on me. My feet meandered from the grass to the sidewalk, to the very edge of the highways, to a high bridge over water, to the edge of that very river that sliced through America, the great Mississippi River, flowing far and fast, from the future to the past.

The doctors told me that if he had been a week older, Baby Jules would have been classified as a stillbirth. They called him a miscarriage. I thought of the medical definition of the word: a spontaneous loss of a fetus before the twentieth week of pregnancy. I kept thinking there was nothing spontaneous about what I had experienced. Spontaneous in the world of writing signifies a surprise, an intervention, a positive impulse. My world of writing had nothing to do with the world I was living in anymore.

In the days after, we went through our lives, a piece at a time, looking for the parts that could hold him, a ghost baby, a dream baby, a baby that was but never will be.

I looked at autumn, my favorite season, as I had never seen it before, barren, full of bold promises waiting to die. Words made no more sense.

My annual garden, dollar-store pots full of cheerful blooms, my geraniums, marigolds, begonias, impatiens, could continue living, but I didn't want them to. I stopped watering them. I watched them die. The blooms withered first, then the leaves started drying out in the sun and the strong winds. I thought about watering them in those final days, but my heart was so heavy I could not find the strength. What did a few more days of bloom matter when in the end, we would all die anyway?

The autumn passed between moments of life feeling almost normal, me talking to the people I love who loved me, trying to find perspective, and then other moments when I wished I had never met my husband and fallen in love with him, gotten married, gotten pregnant, when I wished I had never delivered a dead baby into the world—a baby the world would never know as mine. Then, I would cry and cry and cry until there were no more tears, until the throbbing in my head grew stronger than the beat of my own heart.

I went outside in cold November. I looked upon my dead plants, pots full of earth and debris, spiderwebs where once petunias had bloomed. Small snowflakes started falling from the gray skies. The cold air cooled the heat in my chest. I breathed deep and watched as the white flakes began covering the world, bit by bit.

My birthday was in December. I could not get up. I was so tired, deep in my bones, detached from the earth. I felt I was on water, floating in some dead sea. My husband insisted I take a pregnancy test. I complied only because I did not have the will to argue.

I was pregnant that December.

That next year, in the month of August, a little girl entered my life. She who would say in moments of courageous defiance and assertion, "I am your firstborn." And I, who love her more than the life I had before her, would speak of a little boy who was once born to me but could not join her in life. Once my words had dissipated in the air around us, her warm hands in mind, her round eyes on my face, I would agree: Yes, Shengyeng, you will always and forever be my very first daughter.

I was pregnant two Decembers after that.

In the great ironies of life, I was pregnant with identical twins, a situation that the doctors assured me was also spontaneous, for there was no medical rhyme or reason to an egg splitting.

By late August, two little boys had entered my life. Their flesh was full, and their bones were heavy, and they grew like weeds in the garden of my love, watered by my tears and my laughter. When Yuepheng and Thayeng learned to talk and they spoke of brothers, they referred only to each other, but in my heart I heard the faint echo of a response from far away, Baby Jules.

From somewhere in the high heavens, the places I could not see, well beyond my gaze, there was a future floating down. Even after Baby Jules died, I was alive, feet on the earth, so I could not outrun that future, and slowly it covered me up.

...

It ends with a love story.

I imagine some day in the far, far future. The movie will have played itself out, the story told. I will be an old woman, and I will sit by some window somewhere. Outside it will be cold. Outside it will be hot. Spring will have become summer, summer will have turned into fall, and then it will be winter at long last.

I imagine I will be warm, a blanket over my lap, a book folded nearby. The space beside me will be empty. The valley of my heart will be full of everything that had transpired in August, the month of my marriage, the month where my baby boy died, the month where my daughter and my sons were born. In the winter of my life, I will remember the space of that hot month. I will remember the young man who was once my lover and my friend, my husband, who came to me bald despite the fact that his face was plump with youth. I will remember my precious little boy made of light and air, a reminder of love eternal. I will remember in the quiet of my heart the sounds of the living, of my daughter and my sons, their stories unfolding in a chorus of words, of laughter and tears—amplified by the microphone of time, sending me off toward the window in the high ceiling, that pathway of starlight and moonlight, made only of love that will lead me toward the land of my ancestors.

Either Side

Chue Moua, with Kao Kalia Yang

I am well beyond my childbearing age now. I have had my children. There are equal numbers on either side: seven living and seven dead.

I started out lucky. The young never know this in the moment, but I'm far from my youth now and can see the memories clearly.

We didn't live long then. Most of the people I knew were dead. We were in the aftermath of a war. We were the remnants of the war, the ones running from the bullets still, this time coming only from the other direction. We were Hmong in the jungles of Laos after the American war had ended, and we were being prosecuted and persecuted for having helped the Americans in the war.

Everything I knew about being a mother I had left behind at the age of sixteen when I made the decision to walk toward marriage with Bee, when I left my mother behind to become a wife. I was sixteen years old, more girl than woman. A few months into my marriage, I was pregnant. My belly ballooned in front of me, and I knew a child was flowering in my womb.

When that baby unfurled her limbs and unleashed her cry on a still March morning, in the misty valley of an enemy village, in the absence of her father, far away from my mother, I knew I would never be the same again. It was my first experience of falling in love on sight. Her eyes were small, her mouth was open wide, her hands and her feet were pink and bare, she wrestled and wiggled toward my bosom, and the unbearable pain I had just undergone, the ache in my back, the need to push, the rupture of flesh and blood, the shifting of bones—all of this dissipated in the wave of love that washed over me.

My firstborn was my best friend, my trusted companion, a vehicle for my joy and my wonder, my hopes and my dreams. She was the reason why I survived the months away from Bee, our run in the jungles of Laos, the crossing of the Mekong River, and life on the shores of Thailand. Much of my life was driven by a desire to protect, to love, and to live with her.

My secondborn was a reminder in the refugee camps of Thailand of what the world could deliver, even in a hard life: someone full of softness. Her fine hair was the color of the golden grass that waved on the faraway hillsides surrounding the camp. Her hands held fast to my fingers, and in their hold I felt the beat of a bird's heart. She was born with wings that allowed her to soar high above the place of our captivity.

My experience of motherhood began gently—for all that I lived in worlds full of fear and death. For this, I am thankful to have received the sweet blessings of life.

What happened after is like a flood. I was heavy with my girls on my arms, their hands layered over my heart. I could not have prepared for what would happen. For the first, the second, the third, the fourth, the fifth, and the sixth child that I lost, or as the Americans call it: miscarried. In Hmong we call it *nchuav menyuam*, to spill children. It does not matter what language we are expressing in, it is the language of loss, the language of almost but never, the language of forever and ever.

The six miscarriages that happened in Thailand happened all in a row. They happened at a time when I did not have much food, when my body was so thin the wind blew me into a curve of bones, a hollow bow around my belly, always burgeoning with life, unable to hold it safely inside. Each of the babies came out sometime in the middle of the journey. They were dead upon their arrival. All were formed enough so that we could tell they were baby boys. All of them were thin and wet, slippery like fish. They came in waves of pain that reminded me I was alive, each in turn, reminding me of the price I had to pay to be alive.

How do I describe the experience now, nearly thirty years after the fact? I was young and I was hopeful. I was poor and I had two living girls to care for. I was with a man who loved me enough but was also learning how to love himself and live a life where he would never be everything he was afraid to aspire toward. We were Hmong refugees living on borrowed land, given food three days a week, expected to wait out the years, a day at a time, for a possibility of a life somewhere we'd never been. Already divorced from the time when I had been a girl, I had become a woman full of the traumas of the war and the happenings in the confines of the camp. I was a woman without options, a woman who had made a decision long ago to choose life—no matter what—and who had to live in the travesty of that truth.

I was a woman who gave up on herself some time in the space of those losses, a woman who tried to kill herself—even with her beautiful daughters and her husband by her side—because she could not look upon a life where she was the source of so much death.

I had gotten into a fight with Bee the night before. We were fighting so much to stay together, to stay in love, to stay alive in those years so full of nothing. My girls were sound asleep, sound in their father's love. The fight must have been stupid, because I don't remember it now, but then all I felt was the eruption in my heart.

I woke up early the next morning in a gray dawn. It had rained in the night, and the earth was wet. The door to our sleeping quarters that we had cracked open after our fight to air out our love carried the flower blooms from faraway places to my nose. In the gray, I saw my husband, his arm stretched across the bodies of our sleeping children, a cover against the night, the cold, and the camp. In the early morning, I put my cold feet on the damp earth and slipped them into my flip-flops.

Outside, most of the camp was still asleep. The early roosters crowed their morning calls. Hungry dogs lurked in the shadows between the houses. I knew only the early morning merchants were up and on their way to the camp market.

I knew that at the market they sold packets of pills that fizzed in water. The pills were used to fizz up water to clean silver. Silver that I didn't own . . . silver like the traditional Hmong necklace that my mother had given me when I married Bee, a prized possession that I lost in the Mekong River on the night of our crossing, because I held tighter to my child than the token of my life as someone's.

As I walked to the water jar near the landing of the shared patio to brush my teeth and comb my hair, I was quiet and dreamy. My steps were unsteady on the stairs. They felt weak. I had just had a miscarriage the week before. Which one? I no longer know. All I recall is that I felt pale, bloodless, and cold. The cold was something I carried in my heart. At the water jar, I brushed my teeth with the cold water, washed my face with a wet towel, and combed my long black hair with a plastic comb. I secured the thick strands in a bun at the back of my head with a hair clip. Then, I stood very still. I waited for a few minutes for some other family member to get up, to hear perhaps Bee call out my name, or one of my daughters murmur for me in her sleep, but that morning there was nothing but the quiet of a world that would continue with or without me.

I could see the grave mounds of Hmong people on the faraway hills, the men and women and children who had died naturally, died from sickness, or died because they had killed themselves, bare places among the green grass. It felt to me that they were the only ones at home in this temporary place, the ones who weren't leaving, the ones who would defy the governments of the world who had told us that we were refugees, that we belonged to no nation, that we were people floating far in the hopes of finding a home. I smiled at the defiance of the dead. I smiled at my own rebellion in response to the life I had been living. I was at peace with the task

I had set before myself—because I believed this is what the world wanted of me.

I thought about the babies I had lost, each in turn, a sliver of a life, the size of a cob of corn, the length of a banana, the width of a cup of tea. I thought about how each had died inside of me. My womb had become a casket. I thought about how each had been buried somewhere, free from ceremony or ritual, from the greetings and goodbyes we granted those who had lived, who had been loved. I understood there was no room in my poverty for that kind of goodbye. I felt that I could not survive another goodbye.

I took careful steps on the slippery earth toward the road that led to the market. My flip-flops were attracted to the earth like a magnet. Raising first one foot, then the next was hard. But I persisted.

I thought most about my mother on that walk to the market to the stall of the old woman who sold the silver-cleaning pills I'd seen many times before. My mother whom I remembered then as an old woman only because I was too young to understand the process of age. My mother who had loved me gently and well, who had given me on my wedding day the best of everything she owned, who had told me not to forget her, who had said, her voice shaking, "When you have your own children, you will understand how much I love you, how much I will miss you."

It was the thoughts of my mother that made the tears in my heart surface on my face. I was sorry I could not return to her alive and well, my children around me, laughing and loving. I knew that I was about to commit the biggest crime against her. How many times had she offered herself on the altar of death so that I might live? After my father died, she had looked upon my brothers and sisters and me and told us not to be afraid, promised us that she would protect us. After the Americans left and when the Communist Pathet soldiers entered our village looking to deliver death, it was she who had said, "Kill me before you kill my children." And now, I would be killing myself. The thought of her disappointment, her anger, her loss drew the water from my eyes, and I unleashed my tears in a fine fall from my eyes.

A cool wind blew when I stood before the old woman at the stall. From the veil of water in my eyes, I saw that she smiled at me in greeting. Her mouth soft and pink. Her gums were bare.

She asked, "What can I get you today, Young Woman?"

I had never been a good liar. I turned my gaze toward the little packets of pills laid out on her table. I knew the truth was in my eyes, in the wash of tears on my face, but I didn't know which tiny plastic bag contained the pills I was looking for, so I looked lost.

I said, "I am looking for silver-cleaning pills."

She answered, "I don't have any."

I had not expected her response.

I raised my gaze, "Please help me?"

Her smile disappeared, and she said, "I will not sell you any silver-cleaning pills today."

I blinked the blurry from my eyes.

I asked, "What other vendors carry the pills?"

She said, "I don't know. It is a long line from here to the end. You walk and you ask them. This old lady does not have any for you today."

I had somehow thought that death would be easy, for all of my life had been hard, and it was death that I had been running from the whole time. Now that I was ready for the encounter, this old woman was not going to help me, she was going to make it hard for me.

I said, "I don't know what you mean."

I could see her clearly now. The white strands in the hair fell from her bun. I could see her brown face, deep crevices of folded flesh, those steady, clear eyes looking upon me with concern.

My hands, which had been cold, griped the corners the rickety table before me, a table filled with tiny packages of pain killers, herbal packages, boxed remedies, soap, toothbrushes, toothpastes, shampoos, conditioner, everything a person may need in the course of life. I leaned toward the woman. She leaned toward me. Her old woman's hands fell atop of mine. They were warm and dry. Our heads were close when she said, "I don't know whose daughter you are or whose wife or whose mother, but you will not be buying silver pills from me on this day."

The tears that had just dried began suddenly again, earnestly. The rain that had drizzled on the walk became a storm of liquid I could not contain. My throat clamped. My hands fisted in a last effort at control in the hold of her hands; her brown fingers tightened over mine.

Her voice gentled, "I will not let anyone else sell you silver-cleaning pills today either."

I pulled my hands free.

I said, "You can't do that."

I wiped my tears, and I turned from an offer that was not lost on me. She didn't look like my mother, but she reminded me of her.

Years after, I can still hear her call after me, as I made my way away from her table, "*Me ntxhais . . .*"

I was not her daughter. I could never be.

I walked, tears falling free, from one vendor to the next, asking for silver-cleaning pills, feeling her gaze on my back the whole time. I defied her the way I used to defy my mother. By the time I reached the end of the line of vendors, I had only three capsules in my hands. None of the women would sell me any. A lone man had sold me three. He said they were his last three.

Beside a grove of sugarcane, in a corner of the camp, I sat by myself on a flat rock. I did not want to be found dirty and wet, just dead. I had nothing to drink the pills down with. I had become too emotional. I wiped the tears from my eyes. I redid my bun at the back of my hair, cognizant that the early morning had left, and if I did not hurry, I would be found before the work could be done. I walked back to the market in a hurry. The slippery mud clung to my flip-flops. The romance of the morning was gone. I was suddenly exhausted. In my exhaustion, I fell. I lost one of the pills in my hands. When I got myself up, I could feel the wet of my sarong clinging to my legs. I had no more patience for me. I walked to the vendor with the drinks, my flip-flops a mess of mud, and bought a sweet drink, one of those syrupy drinks that my children liked, the kind that came from a plastic bag with a straw tucked at one end. On my way back to the sugarcane grove, I downed the drink and the two pills I had left. I sat on the rock, I raised my legs and wrapped my arms around my knees, and I laid my tired head to rest.

I understand that a child came upon me first and screamed. Bee said that he had been looking for me. The wet earth had given him a clean track to follow. I wasn't meant to die that morning. Bee said when he heard the child scream in fear, he was already close. By the time, he got to me, there was fizz coming out of my mouth. My eyes were rolled back. I had toppled on the ground.

I woke up at the camp hospital. I heard the whirl of the fan over me. For a moment, I thought I had had another miscarriage. Another child had spilled from me. Bee was where he usually was, sitting beside me, his head in his hands. I closed my eyes again because I did not want to talk or be talked to. I felt very much my own childishness then. I was in my early twenties. I was shy and embarrassed. I pretended to be unconscious for much longer than I was, but I could not pretend forever.

Soon enough, I had to ask about my children, not the ones who had died, but the ones who were alive.

Soon enough, I had to hear my husband's cries and my own in response, first halting and quiet, and then loud, full of the ache inside of me.

Soon enough, I must have gotten pregnant again, and soon enough I must have lost the next baby and the next.

There were points where I decided we would stop trying.

There were points where Bee decided we would stop trying.

But always, in the aftermath of the conversations, the decisions, the declarations we made to each other of our love, we were swept up in our own seas of despair. Neither of us was willing to do the one thing it would take to ensure that we wouldn't conceive again: leave each other.

I had six miscarriages all in a row in the space of the eight years we lived in Ban Vinai Refugee Camp. Sometimes, I know the number is so high that when I say it, other women are not sure how to feel, or how to respond, so I don't say it often, but when asked about why we had only two girls or if we wanted boys, I always answered truthfully. I would not deny the fact that I had tried. I've rarely spoken of what it has cost me to try and try again.

In America, we dreamt that perhaps we would have a successful pregnancy, but we were also full of fear, so we did not speak our dreams aloud to others or to each other. But in America, even without words, there was enough food to keep my belly full and my blood thrumming. In America, I got pregnant again, and again, and again. I had five more live births. One, like the ones in Thailand, a miscarriage halfway in between the string of living children.

Of all the miscarriages I have had, it is perhaps that one in America that traumatizes me the most. It happened in the middle of those years, between the two live births before, and the two after. It was a little boy, also. This time, I knew the size of an American bottle. This time, I knew he would have lived. If it had not been for an American doctor who'd prescribed a medication I was not supposed to be on, if it had not been me, a Hmong woman who could not tolerate a small itch on her skin, so she returned and returned again to the American doctor.

I had developed an itch on my neck. It would eventually be diagnosed as a sun allergy, but then it was just this itch that would not go away. I visited the American doctor, a woman I liked just fine, and she prescribed topical creams that I used to no avail. I returned to see her. She prescribed increasingly stronger medication. Still, it did not work. Finally, she wrote a prescription for a pill that was supposed to make the itch go away.

I had just returned home from work at the factory. My jeans were tight around my middle. I'd long taken off the belts I wore to keep the jeans fitted. My belly was growing. At home, a sink full of dishes waited for me.

The two older girls were at their homework. Bee was gone on the night shift. My little baby boy and girl played on the ground, laughing and rolling around. I changed out of my work clothes, and I put on soft cotton pajamas. I was tired that day, but like all the days before and after there was no place for rest. I washed the dishes at the sink. I complained a little to the older girls. They knew better. I needed more help around the house. In my irritation, I felt the itch at my neck was particularly bad, so I scratched and scratched. Before I took the pill, I made sure to eat a banana. I didn't want an upset stomach. The pill bottle was hard to open, but I managed. I did not read the label. I saw only my name on it. I took the pill with a mug of warm water. I settled on the sofa with my younger two.

That night, I felt a cramp. I could not find a comfortable position between my two youngest on our queen-sized mattress in our small, cramped room. I heard when Bee came home in the early morning hours. I did not call him, because I didn't want to wake up the sleeping children on either arm. When Bee came into our room and saw that I was not yet asleep, he asked if I was alright. I told him that I felt cramps. He asked if I wanted to go to the hospital. I said no. He told me to wake him up if things got worse. They didn't. I was still up when my alarm for work sounded. I got up carefully from the space I occupied, a tiny sliver of bed now that Bee was sleeping, too, clinging to his edge of the mattress. In the bathroom, I saw myself, and there was a look on my face that I recognized, the old defeated look I'd seen in my eyes long ago. I knew my baby had died.

I sat in the darkened house, and I waited for my two older daughters to get up. When they saw me on the sofa, still in the soft pajamas of the night before, they asked, "Niam, are you okay? Are you going to work today?"

I said I wasn't. I said I didn't feel good. I was waiting for their father to get up. They wanted to know if I wanted them to wake him up.

I said, "No. It is alright."

They got ready for school. They kissed me as they headed out the door.

When Bee woke up to find me at the sofa in the same place, he asked again, "What's wrong?"

I told him we needed to drop off the younger kids at his brother's house. I told him that we had to go to the hospital. I told him that I was worried that my baby was dead.

He asked no questions. We moved quickly as a team. The little ones were still tired and made no fuss in our arms as we gathered them into the car.

On the drive to Bee's brother's house, he drove with his left hand and kept his right hand on my hand. He squeezed my hand periodically. We did not have much to say to each other. It was all too familiar, and yet somehow had become so different. We were older now. We'd survived the war in Laos, the refugee camps of Thailand, and were making a go at the poverty we inhabited in America. This time, we knew we would make it through this, and somehow that knowledge made losing the baby worse.

At the hospital, the people did what they were supposed to do, and we followed their instructions. We signed in and showed them our insurance card. Bee and I both expressed in English that we were worried about the baby inside of me. The nurses and doctors nodded their understanding. They moved us from the waiting room into an exam room. They took out the Doppler machine. Different technicians had a listen to the quiet baby inside of me. Different doctors came in, and they pressed into my belly with gloved fingers, then they had me moved into a fancier room with more computers. They looked at the baby inside of me via ultrasound. They were sad when they pronounced that the baby was dead inside of me. But none of the people in the room, not even Bee, none of the people in this whole wide world, was as sad as I was.

The way I was sad about this miscarriage was similar to the sadness I felt when I heard that my mother had died in Laos, far away from me, when my sister told me the news of her death over the hanging phone in the kitchen of that haunted house we lived in for a time. It was this thing that sucked the air out of my chest. It was the kind of sad that you feel when you have to say goodbye to someone who had loved you for a great long time but you knew you could never love them in return in the same way, a debt you would always owe.

What happened after, despite the fact that this time we were in America and all those other times we were in the refugee camps of Thailand, was all too familiar. The baby came out, and it was a boy. His eyes were closed, and his hands were fisted. His body was the size of a bottle. I thought about this all the time—in the days, weeks, months, years after whenever I fed my little ones at home with a bottle. I found myself, late in the quiet of the night and early as the fingers of the sun began to slip into the heavy skies, holding the bottle the way I would have held my baby—if he had been alive.

It will take me the rest of my lifetime to meet him again.

My journey as a mother has been long, continues to be long. When you have seven living on this side and seven waiting on the other side, either place feels like it could be home. I know this is not what many people want to hear, but it is the way my life has turned out to be. It is my experience of loving across the divide of life and death. I've ventured far to be here. I'll venture far to be there. I've tried to make that journey before, so I know: nothing is easy, nothing is close, anywhere is everywhere when you are perpetually looking for a mother's love, looking to be a mother with endless love.

Thirteen Ways of Looking at a Miscarriage

Sun Yung Shin

The poem's form and all italicized text are borrowed from "Thirteen Ways of Looking at a Blackbird" by Wallace Stevens.

I

Among the roving fields inside my body
The only moving thing
Was the sound of my listening.

II

I was of several minds
Like a mother
A body like a waiting room, or a morgue.

III

Some rain gathered in some inner horizon
It was a small part of where the sky met a flood inside me.

IV

A man and a woman
Are one.
A man and a woman and a miscarriage
Are (n)*one.*

V

I do not know which to prefer,
The emptiness of fullness
Or the fullness of emptiness—
The child named before
Or never *after.*

VI

Time *filled the long window*
With *unfinished* glass.
The shadow of the not-child
Cut it like a cord
The organ
Traced in the shallows
In silence, *an indecipherable cause.*

VII

O unfinished child,
Did *you imagine* my face?
Did you not know of the seas
That multiplied around your eye-spot
Lightless as your room?

VIII

I know what it is to "give birth"
And lucid, inescapable rhythms;
Now *I know, too,*
That death is a kind of birth
In what I know.

IX

When you *flew out of sight,*
You left an illegible trail
Where I could not follow.

X

At the sight of your permanent absences
Taken up residence
In the invisible carriage behind me
I became the twin horses of fruitless labor.

XI

What is ten weeks
In a glass coach.
No one told me I would convulse
And pulse blood
Until the glass coach burst
Even *the shadow* of my blood
Made of blood.

XII

The river is moving.
The carriage *must be* sent on.

XIII

It was evening all afternoon.
It was evening all year.
And the years after.
Every month, my blood remembers
How to pour itself, as from a glass.

Acknowledgments

It has been gray for days in Minnesota. The mornings are layered with dark clouds, the sky so full and heavy that it falls low to rest on the earth. In the auspices of dawn, in the early breaths of a new day, highways and school-yards, our very homes, become the backdrop to anything and anywhere at all.

The children we know and love reach out to us with ghostly hands from the places where we dream and the places where our dreams turn into life.

Nearly a year since we started, we are putting together the final words to *What God Is Honored Here?* We have grown older and wiser since this journey began in a different year, on a different day, in a moment where the sky and the earth were divided by a banner of loneliness, a width of invisible space that held us each tight in our bubbles of grief. Now we stand, sisters on earth, looking up at all the bubbles of our lost loves floating high above our heads, trying to feel for the direction of the wind, hopeful that the possibilities within those bubbles, now clad in the words of their mothers, will travel far beyond all of us.

This book has been a blessing of friendship and sisterhood, of solidarity and solace as we welcomed the stories of the women in this collection into our hearts and our homes. This book has been a gift.

To the women who shared their stories of miscarriage and infant loss with us: we are grateful. Your bravery is both inspiring and healing.

To the people at the University of Minnesota Press, particularly Erik Anderson, our editor: you made a difficult journey smooth, paved the hard ground so we could travel without the hurts that are so often a part of this industry.

To all the women out there waiting for this book and finding it in the world: we were always writing for you first. You are our imagined sisters and our dear friends in this journey of womanhood, forces of joy and sorrow, brave spirits carrying forth life and love, even in the face of heartbreaking loss.

To our families: we are so lucky to be loved and supported by you on this adventure that is our life together.

From Shannon: Thank you to Boisey, Sianneh, and Marwein, for always grounding me in this life, and in time and space, and for guiding me and teaching me to continue to open, share, and learn, even when it is very difficult. Thanks to all Sister Friends, family, and community far and near for taking care of me when I could not take care of myself; special thanks to Bobbi Chase Wilding, Taiyon Coleman, Kathleen DeVore, Shalini Gupta, Juliana Hu Pegues, Jae Ran Kim, Sue Gibney, Jim Gibney, Dagny Hanner, and Karen Hausdoerffer. Thanks to the midwife team at Health Foundations for going above and beyond, and standing with me through it all.

From Kalia: Thank you to Thayeng, Yuepheng, Shengyeng, and Baby Jules, for the softness you offered in the gift of having been part of me, for the grace you give in the face of my mistakes, and for living my truths and my tragedies, for being—always—my dearest reminders of why this life matters and means so much for the future. Thank you to my mother, whose life story teaches me who and how I can be in the face of tremendous hardship and pain, who frees me up from judgment so I can experience the fullness that is life without misgivings or regret.

ACKNOWLEDGMENTS

From these long days when the earth has lost its color and the wind has grown cold, from the days of dreaming of warmer weather and the good times still to come.

Kalia in St. Paul and Shannon in Minneapolis
January 15, 2019

Contributors

JENNIFER N. BAKER is a publishing professional, creator and host of the Minorities in Publishing podcast and contributing editor to *Electric Literature*. She works with the nonprofit I, Too Arts Collective and is a 2017 NYSCA/NYFA Artist Fellow and Queens Council of the Arts New Work Grant winner. She is editor of *Everyday People: The Color of Life—A Short Story Anthology* and has published in *Newtown Literary* (her story was nominated for a Pushcart Prize), Longreads, and *Poets & Writers* magazine, among other print and online publications. Her website is jennifernbaker.com.

MICHELLE BOROK is a Korean American writer living in Darkhan, Mongolia, with her husband and daughter. She moved to Mongolia from Los Angeles in 2012. She has written about her life in Mongolia for *Giant Robot, Roads & Kingdoms,* and other arts and culture websites.

LUCILLE CLIFTON (1936–2010) was a prolific poet and author. She served as the Poet Laureate of Maryland from 1979 to 1985. In 1988, two of her books, *Good Woman: Poems and a Memoir, 1969–1980* and *Next: New Poems,* were nominated for the Pulitzer Prize, making her the first author to have two books of poetry chosen as finalists in the same year. In 2000, she was awarded the National Book Award for Poetry for her collection *Blessing the*

Boats: New and Selected Poems, 1988–2000. In 2007 she won the prestigious Ruth Lilly Poetry Prize, which honors a living U.S. poet whose "lifetime accomplishments warrant extraordinary recognition."

SIDNEY CLIFTON is the daughter of the late poet Lucille Clifton. She provides mentorship to young artists from her experience as an Emmy-nominated producer, director, executive producer, video game and animation studio recruiter, writer, speaker, and animation studio executive.

TAIYON J. COLEMAN is a Cave Canem and VONA fellow. Her writing has been published in *Bum Rush the Page, Riding Shotgun, The Ringing Ear, Blues Vision, How Dare We! Write: A Multicultural Creative Writing Discourse,* and *A Good Time for the Truth: Race in Minnesota.* "Mapping Our Potential: A Poem as a Spatial and Temporal Mapping of Human Experience" is her TEDx talk. Her book *Working toward Racial Equity in First-Year Composition* was published in 2019. She is assistant professor of English literature at St. Catherine University in St. Paul, Minnesota.

ARFAH DAUD was born in Malaysia but has made California her home. She began writing more than twenty years ago, after her children were grown. Her work has been published in *Susan B and Me, Byzantium, The Mom Egg, Spillway, Sin Fronteras, New Plains Review, SoloNovo, Apple Valley Review,* and *Watershed Review.* Her poem "Looking Back" was nominated for Best New Poets, Best of the Net, and the Pushcart Prize. She lives in Santa Cruz, California, where she teaches high school.

RONA FERNANDEZ is a writer, fund-raiser, activist, dancer, wife, and #stillmother who lives in the San Francisco Bay Area. Her writing has been published in the *Devilfish Review, Philippine News, The Rumpus, Yes! Magazine,* and other publications. She is an alumnus of the VONA Voices

Workshop for writers of color and the Macondo Workshop. She is grateful to her husband, Henry, for his ceaseless support of her writing. You can find more of her writing at ronafernandez.com.

SHANNON GIBNEY is a writer, educator, and activist. Her first novel, *See No Color*, drawn from her life as a transracial adoptee, won a Minnesota Book Award, as did her second novel, *Dream Country*, which chronicles five generations of a Liberian and Liberian American family. She lives in Minneapolis with her children.

SARAH AGATON HOWES is an Anishinaabe mother, artist, designer, teacher, and community organizer from the Fond du Lac Reservation in Minnesota. She is recognized across the region for her contemporary Ojibwe design and for teaching Makazinikewin (moccasin making). She is an Inspired Native Collaborator creating Ojibwe floral design through her business House of Howes. Her writing is an attempt to convey her raw truth and her grandmother's truth, and to elevate the truths of Indigenous people.

HONORÉE FANONNE JEFFERS is a fiction writer, poet, and critic. Her essays, poems, and short stories have been published in *Angles of Ascent: A Norton Anthology of Contemporary African American Poetry*, *Callaloo*, *The Fire This Time: A New Generation Speaks about Race*, *Iowa Review*, *The Kenyon Review*, *Poetry*, *Prairie Schooner*, *Shenandoah*, and *Virginia Quarterly Review*. She has written four poetry volumes, most recently *The Glory Gets*. She has received fellowships from the Aspen Summer Words Conference, the Bread Loaf Writers Conference, the National Endowment for the Arts, and the Witter Bynner Fellowship through the Library of Congress, as well as an award from the Rona Jaffe Foundation and the Harper Lee Award for Literary Distinction, a lifetime achievement award. She is critic-at-large for *The Kenyon Review* and teaches at the University of Oklahoma.

SONIAH KAMAL is an award-winning essayist and fiction writer. Her debut novel, *An Isolated Incident,* was a finalist for the Townsend Prize for Fiction, and the KLF French Fiction Prize. *Unmarriageable: Jane Austen's Pride and Prejudice in Pakistan* is a *People* Magazine's Pick, a Library Reads Pick, and an Amazon Best Books Pick. Her TEDx talk, "Redreaming Your Dream," is about regrets, second chances, and redemption. Her writing has been published in the *New York Times,* the *Guardian, BuzzFeed,* and *Literary Hub.* Visit her at www.soniahkamal.com.

DIANA LE-CABRERA is a first-generation Vietnamese woman and ever-dreamer. Her parents instilled a passion for learning and creativity early. She earned her master's degree in health sciences, and her work experience is with people of all ages across various industries, from health care to tech to education. Married to her love, Luis Cabrera, she is grateful for her family and hopes to make their children proud.

JANET LEE-ORTIZ is a mother of three: her sunshine, her angel, and her long-awaited rainbow. Her husband is a stay-at-home father and an incredible life partner. Her primary passion is education; she has served as a teacher in Los Angeles Unified School District since 2003. She is a fierce advocate for social justice and engages in activism as a mother. Her hobbies include soccer, snowboarding, hiking, family travels, Korean drumming, and blogging and vlogging. After struggling with fertility, at the time of this writing the family was welcoming the newest member of their family—a daughter.

JAMI NAKAMURA LIN is a Chicago-based writer and library assistant. She has received an inaugural Walter Dean Myers Grant from We Need Diverse Books and a Creative Artists' Fellowship from the National Endowment of the Arts and the Japan–U.S. Friendship Commission. Her stories and essays have been published in *The Baltimore Review, Passages North, [PANK], Bat City Review,* and other publications. She received her MFA in creative

nonfiction from The Pennsylvania State University. Her website is jami
nakamuralin.com.

MARIA ELENA MAHLER'S poems and short stories are published inter-
nationally in English and Spanish journals and anthologies. Her first
bilingual poetry collection, *Sweeping Fossils,* was published in 2016. She
was a finalist for the 2011 San Francisco–based Primer Concurso de Poesía
Latinoamericana en Español and a finalist in the BorderSenses poetry
competition in 2015. She coauthored the nonfiction book *The Heart of
Health* and was editor of the poetry anthology *Woman in Metaphor.* She was
raised in the south of Chile and, after living and working in Mexico and
Canada, now resides between the woods of Northern California e o mato
do Brasil.

CHUE MOUA is Hmong American and a refugee from Laos. She is the
mother of seven living children and seven dead. One of the first girls in
her village to attend school, she is among the first Hmong women of her
generation to be literate. She speaks Hmong, Thai, Lao, and some English.
She has spent her life in America in the factories of Minnesota, keeping
pace with the moving assembly lines. A lifelong gardener, she cares for
beautiful flowers in her house across all seasons and a bountiful organic
garden during the summer.

JEN PALMARES MEADOWS earned her master of arts in creative writing
from California State University Sacramento. Her writing has been published in *Literary Hub, The Rumpus, Fourth Genre, Brevity,* and *The Los Angeles
Review.* She is a 2018 Millay Colony Fellow and is completing a hybrid
collection of gambling essays.

In the eight hours for what we will, DANIA RAJENDRA prefers to argue
politics while knitting something deliciously complicated and drinking
something velvety.

MARCIE RENDON is an enrolled citizen in the White Earth Nation. Her debut novel, *Murder on the Red River,* won the Pinckley Women Debut Crime Writers Award and was the Spur Finalist in the Western Writers of America contemporary novel category; it has been followed by the second book in the series, *Girl Gone Missing.* Among her nonfiction children's books is *Pow Wow Summer.* With four published plays, she is the creative mind behind Raving Native Theater productions. She received the Loft's 2017 Spoken Word Immersion Fellowship with poet Diego Vazquez for work with incarcerated women and was honored as one of 50 over 50 in the Pollen/AARP awards in 2018.

SEEMA REZA is a poet and essayist and author of *When the World Breaks Open* and *A Constellation of Half-Lives.* Based outside Washington, D.C., she is executive director of Community Building Art Works, an arts organization that encourages the arts as a tool for narration, self-care, and socialization among a military population struggling with emotional and physical injuries. An alumnus of Goddard College and VONA, her writing has appeared online and in print in *Bellevue Literary Review, The LA Review, The Feminist Wire, The Offing,* and *Entropy.*

신 선 영 SUN YUNG SHIN was born in Seoul, Korea. She is author of the poetry and essay collections *Unbearable Splendor* (winner of a Minnesota Book Award), *Rough, and Savage,* and *Skirt Full of Black* (which received an Asian American Literary Award). She is editor of *A Good Time for the Truth: Race in Minnesota,* coeditor of *Outsiders Within: Writing on Transracial Adoption,* and author of the bilingual illustrated book for children *Cooper's Lesson.* With poet Su Hwang she cofounded and codirects Poetry Asylum, a poetry-centered organization that creates platforms and spaces for marginalized voices, operating under three commitments: all language is political, no one is illegal, and poetry is a human right. She lives with her partner and children in Minneapolis.

KARI SMALKOSKI is the co-founder of Minnesota Youth Story Squad, a University of Minnesota initiative that partners with public schools to amplify the voices of youth. She is author of the forthcoming book *American Dream Disrupted: Reframing Narratives on Asian American Youth, Gender, and Inequality in Schools*. She has worked as a teacher with high school and college-aged youth for almost two decades and is a proud Minneapolis Public Schools parent. Learn more about her work at her website, youthstorysquad.org.

CATHERINE R. SQUIRES is an author and professor at the University of Minnesota. She has published multiple books on the politics of race, gender, and media, including *The Post-racial Mystique* and the edited collection *Dangerous Discourses: Feminism, Gun Violence, and Civic Life*. She lives with her partner and children in St. Paul, Minnesota, where she is always on the lookout for interesting birds.

Philippine-born and LA-raised, ELSA VALMIDIANO is a writer and poet who calls Oakland home. A former reproductive rights activist, she incorporates her activism into her literary endeavors. Her writing has been published in *TAYO*, *make/shift*, *As/Us*, *Literature for Life*, *Mud Season Review*, *Yes, Poetry*, and *Northridge Review*, as well as in the anthologies *Field of Mirrors*, *Walang Hiya*, and *Circe's Lament*. She is an alumna of the DISQUIET International Literary Program in Lisbon as well as Summer Literary Seminars hosted in Tbilisi. She holds an MFA in creative writing from Mills College and has performed readings at Artists Against Rape, Kearny Street Workshop's APATURE, Scriptorium, Litquake, and Lark Poetry Series. You can read more about her work at slicingtomatoes.com.

KAO KALIA YANG is a Hmong American writer. She is author of *The Latehomecomer: A Hmong Family Memoir*, winner of the Minnesota Book Award in creative nonfiction and memoir and Readers Choice, and a finalist for the PEN USA Award in Creative Nonfiction and the Asian Literary Award in Nonfiction. Her second book, *The Song Poet,* also won the Minnesota Book Award in creative nonfiction and memoir, as well as being a finalist for the National Book Critics Circle Award, the Chautauqua Prize, a PEN USA Award in Nonfiction, and the Dayton's Literary Peace Prize. Her first children's book, *A Map into the World*, about refugees in America, is forthcoming.